Allied Health Professions

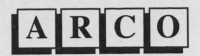

Allied Health Professions

The Arco Editorial Board

Prentice Hall

NEW YORK   LONDON   TORONTO   SYDNEY   TOKYO   SINGAPORE

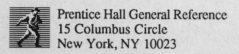 Prentice Hall General Reference
15 Columbus Circle
New York, NY 10023

Copyright © 1993 by Arco Publishing, a division
of Simon & Schuster, Inc.

An Arco Book

Arco, Prentice Hall and colophons are
registered trademarks of Simon & Schuster, Inc.

Library of Congress Cataloging-in-Publication Data

Allied health professions / the Arco Editorial Board
        p.   cm.
ISBN 0-671-84708-2
1. Allied health personnel--Vocational guidance. 2. Allied health personnel--
Examinations, questions, etc. I. Arco Publishing Company.
    [DNLM: 1. Allied Health Occupations. 2. Career Choice. W 21.5
A436 1993]
R697.A4A44 1993
610.73'7--dc20   92-48351
DNLM/DLC   CIP

Manufactured in the United States of America

1 2 3 4 5 6 7 8 9 10

First Edition

Contents

• • • • • • • • • • • • •

PART 3. Information Sources

Introduction

• • • • • • • • • • • • • • •

According to the United States Department of Labor, seven out of ten of the fastest-growing occupations through the year 2000 will be health related. The fields of health care and medical technology are booming today, and the trend is expected to continue. The person who chooses to establish a career in the allied health professions is choosing a lifetime of job security.

Health care encompasses a variety of careers in which health services and technology are the primary concentrations. There are a number of reasons for the growth of this field. The major cause is the tremendous expansion of new technology. Development of advanced equipment in the fields of imaging, laboratory analysis, laser surgery, laparoscopy, and many other areas of instrumentation, along with the explosion of actual knowledge and understanding in medicine, improves quality of life and extends life itself. The extension of life through technology and medicine means that there is a continuing increase in the older population. Elderly people tend to require more medical services, more social services, and more custodial services as they advance in age. The extension of life through medicine and technology also means the survival of many disease and accident victims and of at-risk newborns who might not have survived just a few years ago. These "survivors" tend to require extensive rehabilitative services and, often, long-term institutionalization as well. Finally, as the right to abortion is curtailed, there will be a greater number of severely handicapped children requiring intensive therapy and, often, specialized individual care.

One of the growing trends in health care is providing services for individuals on an outpatient basis. This will create job opportunities for health care practitioners in outpatient clinics, urgi-centers, surgi-centers, mobile offices, schools, and community centers as well as in hospitals. Allied health care professionals will find themselves providing a great many services directly to clients, though of course many will be providing backup services to physicians and institutions as well.

While the outpatient services trend is growing at a tremendous rate, the largest employers of health care professionals will still be hospitals, nursing homes, and extended care facilities. While the role of nursing homes and extended care facilities seems to be most visible in connection with the elderly, the AIDS and tuberculosis crises are adding a new dimension to their use. This is an interesting and exciting time to be entering the health care world.

The book you have in your hands will introduce you to this world. You will begin with an overview of the breadth of the field. While some types of work will probably not interest you at all, other job titles will undoubtedly pique your interest and lead you to investigate ways in which you might fit in. Following the overview, you will find in-depth profiles of twenty-eight selected careers. You will want to read some of these a few times, taking notes and following through on the sources for further information. Others you may skim or skip altogether.

Not every allied health training program requires that you pass an examination for admission, but many do. Part Two includes a full-length sample Allied Health Professions Admission Test with explanations of all the correct answers. If you might be applying to one of the 400 schools that require this exam, you can get good practice. If you must take some other exam, practice with this sample exam, while perhaps not right on target, will be helpful too. If your exam will be the Allied Health Aptitude Test, practice with the sample AHPAT will put you ahead of the game. The AHAT is similar to the AHPAT but somewhat easier in content. Part Three offers you a wealth of information sources. Here you will find an extensive list of societies, associations, and boards, with their addresses and telephone numbers, for information about many allied health careers and training programs. There is also a directory of schools that offer training programs for most of the twenty-eight careers described in detail in Part One.

1

The Careers

The Health Care Field

• • • • • • • • • • • • • • •

The wide range of occupations within the health care field offers many choices to the person who is seeking a career in a health-related profession. From the entry-level, minimal-training positions of Home Health Care Aide or Hospital Orderly to the heavily credentialed Biochemist or Podiatrist or Registered Nurse, there is a niche for nearly every interest and for every degree of skill.

High school graduates can enter the health care world and receive on-the-job training, performing meaningful work from the very outset of their careers. Other high school graduates may enroll in certification programs that give them classroom instruction and supervised field experience so that they are well prepared to take over in specific roles. Certification programs are offered by specialized technical schools, by many hospital schools, and by community and junior colleges. The college-sponsored programs may offer an associate's degree along with the proficiency certificate. Degrees raise earning power. Allied health care professionals often go on to earn degrees while working in their fields. The health care arena is open and flexible, as befits a growing career field. Beyond the associate level, many health care professionals receive their bachelors' degrees at colleges and universities, perhaps in conjunction with professional certification programs such as those for Registered Nurses. And, of course, there are degree-related and skill-related programs that reach beyond the bachelor's level as well.

The beauty of the health care field is that experience gained at entry- and intermediate-level jobs is im-mediately applicable at the next levels. While most intermediate- and upper-level positions will require formal schooling, no task from the lower level will have been a waste of time. Training and experience both help the health care professional on the way up the career ladder.

The following alphabetical list of job titles in the health care world—from entry-level through top-ranked professionals—is lengthy but far from comprehensive. This list should open your eyes to the array of possibilities.

Alcohol and Drug Abuse Counselor

Art Therapist

Audiologist

Biochemist

Biomedical Engineer

Blood Bank Technologist

Cardiopulmonary Technologist

Cardiovascular Perfusion Technologist

Certified Laboratory Assistant

Chiropractor

Circulation Technologist

Clinical Laboratory Technologist

Cytotechnologist

Dance Therapist

Dental Assistant

Dental Hygienist

Dentist

Diagnostic Sonographer

Dietitian and Nutritionist

Dispensing Optician

EEG Technologist/Technician

EKG Technician

Emergency Medical Technician

Genetic Counselor

Geriatric Assessment Coordinator

Geriatric Social Worker

Health Educator

Health Services Administrator

Home Health Aide

Hospital Administrator

Licensed Practical Nurse (LPN)

Medical Assistant

Medical Illustrator

Medical Records Technician

Medical Technologist

Nurse Anesthetist

Nurse's Aide

Nursing Assistant

Nursing Home Activites Director

Occupational Therapist

Optometrist

Orthopedic Assistant

Orthotist

Osteopath

Pharmacist

Psychologist

Physical Therapist

Physical Therapy Assistant

Physician

Physician's Assistant

Podiatrist

Prosthetist

Radiation Therapist

Radiologic Technologist

Recreation Therapist

Registered Nurse (RN)

Respiratory Therapist

Social Worker

Sonographer

Speech Pathologist

Speech Therapist

Surgical Technologist

Veterinarian

Veterinary Technician

We have selected twenty-eight representative allied health careers from the above list and have described these at greater length. In the following pages, you can learn about these careers—the work that is done, the opportunities, the education and experience requirements, and the earnings outlook. The directory of societies, associations, and boards in Part Three can lead you to still more information on these twenty-eight careers and to information on many of the other allied health careers as well.

Twenty-Eight Representative Careers*

• • • • • • • • • • • • • • • • • •

PODIATRIST

. . . .

Job Description: Diagnose and treat foot problems; perform therapy and surgery on feet/lower leg.

Earnings: $35,000 to $150,000+

Recommended Education and Training: Degree from an accredited college of podiatry.

Skills and Personality Traits: Manual dexterity; interpersonal skills; compassion; business skills; proficiency in the sciences.

Experience and Qualifications: State licensing and residency program.

Job Description and Responsibilities

Podiatrists are doctors who treat foot and lower leg conditions. They are responsible for the diagnosis and treatment of abnormalities, injuries, and diseases of this area of the human body.

While podiatry has been a medical specialty throughout the years, it is currently becoming more widely recognized and generally used. As people live longer there is greater wear and tear on all body parts, especially the feet. The popularity of podiatry, even among the younger population, is enhanced by the current interest in health, fitness, sports, and exercise.

To correct foot problems, podiatrists often prescribe special shoes or shoe inserts. Today, podiatrists use computerized machinery that reads the foot size, shape, and exact dimensions to get a perfect fit for a corrective shoe or insert device. Sophisticated equipment of this type will become even more prevalent in the future.

Surgery is a major duty of many podiatrists. Used to correct deformities or problems such as bunions or hammer toes, surgery may be performed in a hospital or in the podiatrist's office.

In many instances, patients make appointments to see podiatrists to have common foot problems treated, such as corns, calluses, or ingrown toenails. Patients may also visit podiatrists for foot or ankle pain resulting

*From the book *100 Best Careers for the Year 2000,* by Shelly Field, © 1992. Used by permission of the publisher: An Arco Book/Prentice Hall/A Division of Simon & Schuster, Inc., New York.

5

from accidents or exercise. A variety of therapeutic procedures and treatments may be used by the podiatrist to heal ailments.

Other functions of podiatrists include diagnosing and treating foot problems that develop as a result of diabetes, heart disease, and other circulatory problems.

Employment Opportunities

Podiatrists may practice in a vast array of settings, including:

- Private practice
- Medical groups
- Hospitals and other health care facilities
- Nursing homes
- Clinics
- Health maintenance organizations (HMOs)
- Public health departments
- Sports medicine clinics

Specialties include:

- Surgery
- Orthopedics
- Primary podiatrics
- Sports medicine
- Public health
- Pediatrics
- Diabetics and other disease-related foot care
- Geriatrics

Expanding Opportunities for the Year 2000

An increase in the popularity of sports, fitness, and exercise will create a demand for podiatrists specializing in sports injuries. A demand will also be seen for podiatrists working with the elderly.

Earnings

Annual earnings for podiatrists can range from approximately $35,000 to $150,000 or more. Earnings are determined to a great extent by the type of situation the podiatrist is working in as well as the experience and reputation of the individual.

Podiatrists who are in private practice in large metropolitan cities and have built good reputations will have earnings on the higher end of the scale. Those who are just starting out will earn considerably less.

Advancement Opportunities

Most podiatrists climb the career ladder by going into private practice. Others advance by specializing in a specific field of podiatry.

Individuals who prefer to be on staff at a facility might locate positions in larger, more prestigious facilities.

Education and Training

Podiatrists must graduate from an accredited college of podiatric medicine. As of now, the only seven states with such schools are California, Florida, Illinois, Iowa, New York, Ohio, and Pennsylvania.

The four-year program includes two years of classroom instruction plus two years of clinical rotation in various practical settings.

After receiving a DPM, or doctor of podiatric medicine degree, most podiatrists go on to a three-year residency program.

In order to be admitted to an accredited college, individuals must complete at least 90 hours of undergraduate study with a good grade point average. Most people who gain acceptance into one of the schools of podiatric medicine, however, have obtained a bachelor's degree prior to their acceptance. Individuals must also obtain a good score on the Medical College Admission Test (MCAT).

Experience and Qualifications

Podiatrists must be licensed in the state in which they work. Licensing requirements, which differ from state to state, usually include graduating from an accredited college of podiatric medicine, passing oral and written examinations, and completing an accredited residency program. In certain states, individuals may take an examination offered by the National Board of Podiatric Examiners in lieu of the state's written examination. Some states may grant reciprocity to individuals licensed in another state.

While podiatrists do not have to be board-certified, it is suggested. The American Board of Podiatric Surgery, The American Board of Podiatric Orthopedics, and the American Board of Public Health all offer certification in their specific specialty.

For Additional Information: Individuals aspiring to be podiatrists can receive additional information from the American Podiatric Medical Association (APMA) or the American Association of Colleges of Podiatric Medicine (AACPA).

TIPS

• If you are just starting your own practice, you might volunteer to be a speaker for meetings of local civic and nonprofit organizations.

• You might find it easier to start a practice in a smaller area in need of a podiatrist rather than in a larger city with a number of practicing podiatrists.

CHIROPRACTOR

Job Description: Perform examinations and therapies; prescribe diets, exercises, and self-care.

Earnings: $40,000 to $180,000+

Recommended Education and Training: Two years of pre-professional college; four years of chiropractic college.

Skills and Personality Traits: Interpersonal skills; sympathy; understanding; communication skills; detail-oriented; manual dexterity.

Experience and Qualifications: State licensing; degree from an approved college of chiropractic.

Job Description and Responsibilities

Chiropractic is based on a holistic view of health care. Chiropractors treat an individual's entire system rather than focusing on just one specific part or patient complaint. They deal with the body's structural and neurological systems, placing special emphasis on the spine. These professionals feel that if any part of the body is misaligned or compressed it can drastically affect the rest of the body and its functions. Chiropractic stresses natural methods of healing without resorting to drugs or surgery.

People go to chiropractors to attain maximum health. Many individuals have either chronic or acute health problems including headaches, backaches, fatigue, and stiff necks. Other patients use chiropractic as a method of preventive health care.

Chiropractors begin by taking a patient's medical history. They find out about previous problems, pains, and discomforts. They also may learn from the history that the patient has been in an accident, fallen, or injured him- or herself in some manner.

Examinations include postural and spinal analysis used in chiropractic diagnosis. They may also include visual, orthopedic, neurologic, or physical examinations; X-rays; and lab tests.

The major treatment used by chiropractors is spinal manipulation and adjustment. Other remedies include various physiological therapies such as water, light, ultrasound, massages, and electric and heat treatments. Many chiropractors counsel patients on stress reduction, nutrition, and exercise. In some instances, chiropractors recommend the use of braces, straps, or other supports to correct body alignment.

Chiropractors who are in their own practice have management duties as well. They may hire and oversee a staff, schedule patients, answer phones, and handle billing and bookkeeping.

Employment Opportunities

Most chiropractors open up their own practice right out of school. Other employment opportunities include:

- Chiropractic clinics
- Working for other chiropractors
- Alternative health care clinics
- Health spas and resorts
- Faculty member of chiropractic college
- Researcher at chiropractic college

Expanding Opportunities for the Year 2000

The growing awareness of chiropractic as an alternative health care system will result in an increased demand for these professionals. Chiropractors have more opportunities for success in small communities where there is little or no competition.

Earnings

Factors affecting earnings include the reputation, experience, personality, geographic location, and marketing skills of the chiropractor. Earnings will also be different for salaried employees than for individuals in their own businesses.

Chiropractors who are salaried may earn between $35,000 and $65,000-plus. Individuals who have their own practices can net between $35,000 and $100,000 or more. Individuals just starting out in private practice will have the lowest earnings. Income will increase as they develop a practice.

Advancement Opportunities

There are a number of ways for chiropractors to advance their careers. Individuals may work for another chiropractor or a chiropractic clinic. After obtaining some experience they may start their own practice. Individuals who are already in their own practice can climb the career ladder by developing a larger patient roster.

Some chiropractors advance by teaching at a chiropractic college or performing research.

Education and Training

Chiropractors must complete two years of college and then the four-year course of study at an accredited chiropractic college.

While chiropractic colleges teach courses in skeletal manipulation and spinal adjustments, there is also a broad range of other courses. The program consists of clinical experience as well as classroom and laboratory work in basic sciences such as anatomy, physiology, chemistry, pathology, hygiene, sanitation, and public health.

Individuals must also take courses in clinical science subjects such as physical, clinical, and laboratory diagnosis; gynecology and obstetrics; pediatrics; roentgenology techniques; geriatrics; dermatology; dietetics; toxicology; and psychology and psychiatry.

Candidates must be at least 21 years old to graduate from an approved college of chiropractic. Those who complete the program are awarded the degree of Doctor of Chiropractic (DC).

Experience and Qualifications

Chiropractors must be licensed in the state in which they work. Many states offer reciprocity. Licensing requirements vary from state to state. Most states require individuals to complete two years of undergraduate education plus four years of chiropractic college at a school accredited by the Council on Chiropractic Education. Individuals must also pass a licensing exam and a basic science examination.

In order to maintain their licenses, chiropractors must take annual continuing education courses.

For Additional Information: For additional information, contact the American Chiropractic Association (ACA), the International Chiropractors Association (ICA), and the Council on Chiropractic Education (CCE).

TIPS

• If you are still in school, consider a part-time or summer job in a chiropractor's office as a secretary or receptionist.

• If you are already in practice, you might offer a free examination or adjustment to new patients.

• If you are just opening up a new practice, volunteer to speak to local civic groups about the chiropractic profession.

REGISTERED NURSE (RN)

Job Description: Care for patients; administer medication; record symptoms; observe progress; supervise LPN's, orderlies, and aides.

Earnings: $21,000 to $55,000+

Recommended Education and Training: Associate degree, bachelor's degree, or diploma from an approved school of nursing.

Skills and Personality Traits: Compassion; desire to help others; reliablity; communication skills.

Experience and Qualifications: State licensing; clinical experience.

Job Description and Responsibilities

Registered nurses have varied responsibilities depending on the setting in which they work. Those working in nursing homes will have different duties than individuals caring for patients in clinics, retirement communities, schools, or other settings. Their main function, however, is to administer medical care to ill or injured individuals.

RN's work beside physicians, assisting in medical care and carrying out the physician's instructions. RN's may be present in the doctor's office when examinations are being conducted and assist in the exam. They take patients' vital signs and may be responsible for taking blood or performing certain laboratory tests. In some instances, they help the physician perform treatments.

Registered nurses working in hospitals or other health care facilities provide the primary bedside nursing care. This includes changing dressings, cleaning wounds, administering medication, starting intravenous fluids, and monitoring medical equipment. RN's also record patients' symptoms and reactions and chart their progress with regard to medication or course of action prescribed by the physician. In some situations they are responsible for assessing needs of patients and developing treatment plans. This is common in nursing homes and extended-care facilities.

A great deal of the work of an RN is administrative or supervisory. Individuals supervise aides, orderlies, and LPN's in their duties. Registered nurses also handle paperwork such as patient charts.

RN's working in schools, prisons, and clinics have various educational duties. They instruct individuals on preventative health care, nutrition, exercise, etc. They also perform various health screenings, tests, and procedures.

Individuals work varied hours depending on the specific employment situation. They are responsible to either the head nurse or the physician in charge.

Employment Opportunities

Registered nurses can work part- or full-time in a variety of health care situations and environments. Some of these include:

- Hospitals
- Health care facilities
- Physicians' offices
- Clinics
- Schools
- Colleges and universities
- Prisons
- Nursing homes
- Extended care facilities
- Health maintenance organizations
- Retirement communities
- Rehabilitation centers
- Health departments of corporations
- Home health care
- Surgi-centers
- Urgi-centers
- Diagnostic imaging centers
- Cardiac rehabilitation clinics

Expanding Opportunities for the Year 2000

There is a shortage of registered nurses in almost all areas and employment settings.

Hospitals and health care facilities can no longer be reimbursed for patients who are hospitalized beyond the normal time for their specific illness. Many patients are, therefore, sent home before they have fully recuperated. This means that there will be a demand for registered nurses who can administer in-home care.

RN's will be in great demand in geriatric settings such as nursing homes and extended care facilities. This is due to the growing older population who require long-term care.

Demand for RN's will be especially high in facilities that care for critically and terminally ill patients.

Earnings

Earnings vary greatly for registered nurses depending on their experience, education, responsibilities, and geographic location. Other factors affecting earnings include the type, size, and prestige of the facility the individual is working in as well as the particular shift.

As a result of the tremendous shortage of RN's, many employers are increasing salaries and benefits to try to lure applicants. Salaries for entry-level RN's range from approximately $21,000 to $28,000. Nurses with more experience may earn up to $45,000 or more with additional training. Those with specialized skills can have annual salaries of up to $55,000.

In addition, most employers offer RN's liberal benefit packages to augment their earnings. Some also offer tuition reimbursement.

Advancement Opportunities

There are many paths to career advancement for registered nurses, depending on the direction they want to pursue. With experience and additional training, individuals may move into supervisory, management, or administrative positions. They may, for example, become the director of nursing of a facility or a head nurse at a clinic. Other RN's seek positions as nurse practitioners, nurse clinicians, nurse anesthetists, or clinical nurse specialists.

Education and Training

Individuals aspiring to become registered nurses may pursue an associate degree in nursing, culminating in an ADN; a Bachelor of Science degree in nursing, called a BSN; or a diploma program. Associate and bachelor's degree programs are offered in community colleges, junior colleges, and colleges or universities. The diploma program is offered by hospitals.

Program length varies. ADN degrees usually require two years of schooling while diploma programs last two to three years. The BSN will generally take four years. Any of the three possible programs will qualify individuals for entry-level positions. However, earnings and advancement will be better for those with BSN's.

Nurses' training includes classroom study, supervised training, and clinical experience. Classes include anatomy, microbiology, chemistry, nutrition, physiology, psychology, nursing, and computer usage.

Experience and Qualifications

Registered nurses must be licensed in the state in which they work. In order to obtain a license, individuals must graduate from an approved school of nursing and pass a national examination administered by the specific state in which they reside. RN's interested in working in another state must either take another examination or be granted reciprocity.

State nursing licenses must be renewed. Some states require continuing education for renewal.

For Additional Information: Individuals interested in becoming registered nurses can obtain additional information by contacting the National Student Nurses' Association (NSNA), the National League For Nursing (NLN), the American Nurses' Association (ANA), the American Hospital Association (AHA), and the American Health Care Association (AHCA).

TIPS

• Many high schools, vocational-technical schools, colleges, and hospitals have health career fairs for people interested in exploring the nursing field.

• Before you make a commitment to nursing, you might want to volunteer in a hospital. This will give you experience in a health care setting. It will also give you an opportunity to see if this type of career is for you.

• Hospitals and other health care facilities often hold teas, luncheons, and dinners to attract new nurses.

• Job openings are advertised in the newspaper classified section under headings such as ''Nurses,'' ''RN's,'' ''Registered Nurses,'' ''Hospitals,'' ''Health Care,'' or the names of specialties.

LICENSED PRACTICAL NURSE (LPN)

Job Description: Perform nursing duties under the supervision of physicians and registered nurses.

Earnings: $13,000 to $30,000

Recommended Education and Training: Completion of a practical nursing program accredited and approved by the state.

Skills and Personality Traits: Compassion; stamina; communication skills; ability to follow directions.

Experience and Qualifications: Experience in a supervised clinical health care setting.

Job Description and Responsibilities

Licensed practical nurses perform a variety of nursing duties under the supervision and direction of physicians and registered nurses. Individuals in this particular field are commonly referred to as LPN's or licensed vocational nurses (LVN's).

No matter what the job title, one of the main functions of an LPN is to make patients as comfortable as possible. LPN's help patients bathe, brush their teeth, and handle other personal hygiene needs.

A major responsibility of LPN's is taking vital signs on a routine basis or at the direction of physicians. Vitals include a patient's temperature, pulse, and blood pressure. The individual must be sure to record the information accurately on the patient's chart.

If an emergency occurs, the LPN should be able to perform CPR (cardiopulmonary resuscitation). Other responsibilities include preparing and administering injections prescribed by a physician. In some instances, where allowed, LPN's will be required to give prescribed medicines to patients. However, not all states allow LPN's to handle this task.

The LPN may work in any unit in the hospital including maternity, intensive care, recovery, skilled nursing, pediatrics, and medical-surgical.

Employment Opportunities

LPN's may work in a number of different health care settings including:

- Hospitals
- Rehabilitation centers
- Nursing homes
- Group homes
- Senior citizen homes
- Extended care facilities
- Physicians' offices
- Clinics
- Private homes (for private duty)
- Temporary nursing agencies

Expanding Opportunities for the Year 2000

There is a great need for LPN's in all health care settings. With new rules and regulations shortening the length of stay patients can have in a facility, there will be a great demand for private duty nurses.

Earnings

Annual earnings for LPN's can range from approximately $13,000 to $30,000. Factors affecting income include the specific facility as well as its size, prestige, and geographic location. Other determining factors include the experience and responsibilities of the LPN.

Advancement Opportunities

Licensed practical nurses may look for career advancement through increased earnings. To accomplish this, individuals can locate similar positions in larger or more prestigious facilities where higher salaries are offered. Others obtain supervisory duties over nursing assistants and nurses' aides.

An LPN might also climb the career ladder by completing the additional education necessary to become a registered nurse.

Education and Training

LPN's must complete a state approved practical nursing program. Generally, in order to enroll in such a program, individuals must be high school graduates. However, there are a number of states in the country that allow candidates into their nursing program after completing one or more years of high school.

Practical nursing programs are usually one year in duration. They are offered through hospitals, community colleges, trade schools, vocational schools, and technical programs. In addition to classroom work, most programs require experience in a supervised clinical setting.

Experience and Qualifications

As noted previously, LPN's must have experience working in a supervised clinical setting. They must also pass a national written examination in order to get their license.

For Additional Information: Individuals interested in becoming Licensed Practical Nurses may contact a number of organizations and associations for more information. These organizations include the National Federation of Licensed Practical Nurses, Inc. (NFLPN), the National League for Nursing (NLN), the National Association for Practical Nurse Education and Service, Inc. (NAPNES), the American Hospital Association (AHA), and the American Health Care Association (AHCA).

TIPS

• Openings for LPN's are usually advertised in the classified section of the newspaper, under headings such as "Nurses," "Licensed Practical Nurses," "LPN's," "Health Care," "Hospitals," "Private Duty," or "Temporary Nursing."

• Send your resume and a short cover letter to the personnel directors of health care facilities. With the shortage of qualified people, you should expect calls for interviews.

• Large cities have employment agencies specializing in jobs in the health care industry.

DENTAL HYGIENIST

· ·

Job Description: Provide preventative dental care; clean teeth; handle curettage.

Earnings: $14,000 to $33,000+

Recommended Education and Training: Graduation from an accredited school of dental hygiene.

Skills and Personality Traits: Personable; good communication skills; compassion; manual dexterity.

Experience and Qualifications: State licensing; graduation from an accredited school of dental hygiene; written and clinical examinations.

Job Description and Responsibilities

Almost everyone has had an opportunity to utilize the services of a dental hygienist during their lifetime.

One of the main functions of most dental hygienists is to clean teeth. Cleaning may be scheduled on an annual, biannual, or quarterly basis, depending on the state of the patient's teeth and gums. The hygienist may also scrape plaque, perform gumline curettage, and apply fluoride or sealers to help retard cavities and plaque build-up. The hygienist will instruct the patient on tooth and gum care and illustrate the correct way to brush and use floss.

Some states allow the hygienist to perform the preliminary examination of the patient's mouth looking for cavities, broken or cracked teeth, gum disease, and oral cancer. The hygienist may also prepare a patient for X-rays and take and develop films.

In certain states, dental hygienists assist dentists in removing sutures, applying dressings, and administering anesthesia, if they have the required education in that specialty.

Dental hygienists may be responsible for keeping records of patient care. They might also schedule appointments, handle billing, answer patient's questions, and run the office.

Dental hygienists may work full- or part-time. In many instances, the individual will work part-time in a number of dental offices. Hours in some offices are very flexible, while others may be the traditional nine-to-five. The hygienist is directly responsible to the dentist in charge of the office.

Employment Opportunities

While individuals may work in a variety of settings, some jobs require additional education. Dental hygienists may work for:

- Private dentist offices
- Group dental practices
- Public clinics
- School systems
- Hospitals
- Dental hygiene schools
- Health maintenance organizations
- Nursing homes
- Extended care facilities
- State health departments

Expanding Opportunities for the Year 2000

As more people become aware of the importance of preventive dental care, there will be a greater demand for dental hygienists in all settings. There will be a special need for hygienists in geriatrics and geriatric facilities as a result of the increase in our aging population.

Earnings

Dental hygienists may be paid by the hour, day, week, or number of patients worked on. Hygienists may also have their salaries augmented by fringe benefit packages.

Individuals working full-time in this profession can have annual earnings ranging from $14,000 to $33,000 or more, depending on setting and job, geographic location, and method of payment. Other factors affecting earnings include the hygienist's education, responsibilities, and experience.

Individuals with the most education and working in large metropolitan cities will have the highest earnings.

Advancement Opportunities

Dental hygienists can advance by locating positions in larger, more prestigious offices. They may also climb the career ladder by obtaining additional education and going after positions in research, teaching, and administration in dental hygiene education programs.

Education and Training

Dental hygienists must graduate from an accredited school of dental hygiene. Areas of study include basic sciences, dental sciences, clinical sciences, and social and behavioral sciences. Laboratory, classroom, and clinical instruction is required.

Hygienists may seek either a two-year associate degree, a four-year bachelor's degree or a master's degree. The two-year degree is usually suitable for working in a private dental office. Four-year or post-graduate degrees are required for positions in teaching, research, clinical practice for public or school health programs, and administrative or teaching positions in dental hygiene education.

Minimum requirements to enter dental hygiene schools vary. There are some programs that prefer or require students to have at least one year of college while others require completion of two years.

Experience and Qualifications

Dental hygienists usually receive practical experience in school. Individuals in all states must be licensed by the state they are working in.

Licensing requirements include graduation from an accredited dental hygiene school and passing both a written and a clinical examination. Individuals may also be required to take another examination on legal aspects of dental hygiene practice.

For Additional Information: Individuals interested in careers in dental hygiene can obtain additional information by contacting the American Dental Hygienists' Association (ADHA), the American Dental Association (ADA), and the American Association of Dental Examiners (AADE).

TIPS

- One of the great things about being a dental hygienist is the flexibility. This is especially important for people who have school-aged children or who are continuing their own education.

- Openings are often advertised in the classified or display section of newspapers under headings of "Dental," "Dental Hygienist," "Dental Office," or "Hygienist."

- If you enjoy working with children, try to locate a pediatric dentist.

- Send your resume and a short cover letter to dentists, clinics, hospitals, and extended care facilities in your area. Request that your resume be kept on file if there are no current openings.

DENTAL ASSISTANT

Job Description: Assist dentist; make patients comfortable; prepare patients for treatment; sterilize instruments.

Earnings: $12,000 to $23,000

Recommended Education and Training: Dental assisting program or on-the-job training.

Skills and Personality Traits: Personable; eager to learn; able to follow instructions; communication skills.

Experience and Qualifications: Some positions require experience; certification available but not required.

Job Description and Responsibilities

Dental assistants work alongside dentists, assisting them in their work. Responsibilities vary depending on the specific job.

Before a dental assistant brings a patient into the dentist's office, the individual will usually prepare for that patient. This may entail cleaning, sterilizing, and disinfecting equipment; preparing a tray of sterilized dental instruments, and getting the patient's chart from the receptionist.

When patients are brought into the treatment room, the dental assistant will try to make them as comfortable as possible in the chair. They will put a bib on the patient to protect their clothing and may inform the dentist that the patient is ready.

When the dentist is working with the patient, the dental assistant will be responsible for passing the specified instruments or materials. The assistant may also use a suctioning device to help keep the patient's mouth dry during procedures.

Dental assistants in some situations take X-rays, remove sutures, apply anesthesia, make casts of the mouth or teeth, or handle other tasks under the direction of the dentist.

In some offices, dental assistants manage the office, schedule and confirm patient appointments, handle billing responsibilities, and maintain records.

Hours are determined by the hours the dentist works. The dental assistant is directly responsible to the dentist.

Employment Opportunities

Dental assistants may work in any setting in which a dentist is at work. These settings include:

- Private dentist offices
- Group dental practices
- Public clinics
- School systems
- Hospitals
- Dental hygiene schools
- Health maintenance organizations
- Nursing homes
- Extended care facilities
- State health departments

Earnings

Salaries for dental assistants working full-time range from approximately $12,000 to $23,000. Factors affecting salary include the specific job and geographical location as well as the experience, education, qualifications, and duties of the dental assistant.

Individuals who have gone through formal training programs and are certified will generally earn more. Salaries will also be higher in areas where there is a special need for dental assistants or in large metropolitan cities where there is a higher cost of living.

Advancement Opportunities

Dental assistants seeking advancement may try to locate similar positions in more prestigious offices.

Individuals who are interested in working in the field of dental hygiene might consider going back to school to obtain the necessary education.

Education and Training

Education and training requirements vary from job to job. In some positions, employers seek individuals who are eager to learn new skills and train them on the job. In others, employers may prefer that their employees go through a formal dental assisting program.

Dental assisting programs are offered throughout the country in vocational, trade, and technical schools as well as in junior or community colleges. Courses of study include classroom, laboratory, and preclinical instruction in dental assisting skills. Many programs also offer practical experience in clinics, dental offices, or affiliated dental schools.

Experience and Qualifications

While some jobs require experience, in most dental offices this is an entry-level position. Certification is available through the Dental Assisting National Board but is not required for most jobs. It does, however, indicate that the individual is competent and may give one person an edge over another. In order to obtain certification, dental assistants must be high school graduates and complete a training program accredited by the Commission on Dental Accreditation or have at least two years of full-time experience as a dental assistant. They must also pass a certification examination and a course in cardiopulmonary resuscitation (CPR).

For Additional Information: Individuals interested in careers in dental assisting can learn more by contacting the American Dental Assistants Association (ADAA), the American Dental Association (ADA), and the Dental Assisting National Board, Inc. (DANB).

TIPS

- Many of the accredited training schools for dental assistants have job placement services.

- Openings may be advertised in the classified or display section of the newspaper. Look under heading classifications for "Dental Office" or "Dental Assistant."

- Write to dentists and dental clinics in the area to find out if they have openings. Remember to send a copy of your resume with a cover letter.

ALCOHOL AND DRUG ABUSE COUNSELOR
· ·

Job Description: Counsel drug or alcohol addicts; run workshops; supervise group therapy sessions; prepare reports.

Earnings: $12,000 to $35,000+

Recommended Education and Training: Educational requirements and training vary from state to state and job to job.

Skills and Personality Traits: Emotional stability; empathy; good interpersonal skills; nonjudgmental; communication skills; ability to work independently.

Experience and Qualifications: Experience depends on job; certification or registration may be required.

Job Description and Responsibilities

Alcohol and drug abuse counselors work with individuals who have addictions or are substance abusers. They may also work with the patients' families. Counselors have varied duties and responsibilities depending on their specific employment situation.

Some patients want to be helped. Others do not. It is often difficult to help patients who do not want to stop substance abuse or do not think they have a problem. It is up to the counselor to develop motivational techniques to move patients through the various steps of therapy.

Alcohol and drug abuse counselors often work with other health professionals including physicians, psychiatrists, psychologists, social workers, and psychiatric nurses. It is up to the counselor to refer patients to the appropriate medical personnel, agency, or program. If the patient must go through detox, it must be done under close medical supervision. Counselors may discuss patients' needs with physicians or nurses assigned to the case.

Counselors may specialize in certain groups of people. For example, they may work only with children or teenagers. Others may counsel business executives. Individuals may also specialize in counseling individuals who abuse specific drugs such as heroin, cocaine,

or alcohol. Special training may be required to work with specific groups.

Alcohol and drug abuse counselors must evaluate and assess each patient separately. They must determine the extent and pattern of an individual's abuse.

Counselors are responsible for providing services to patients and their families. They may work with the patient on a one-on-one basis; with the patient and the family; or in a group counseling situation. During these sessions, they attempt to help the patient to cease using substances. In a group therapy situation, counselors will supervise the group, trying to move it in positive directions.

Counselors ask probing questions and do a great deal of listening. They may do this to evoke certain emotions in the patient and break down psychological walls. Counselors and patients who are in these situations often build a close working rapport.

There is a great deal of paperwork involved in alcohol and drug counseling. Individuals must prepare reports on patients in order to follow their progress. Counselors will often be required to participate in staff team meetings, develop treatment plans, and contribute to the multidisciplinary treatment plan for each patient.

Other duties include assisting with a patient's social welfare needs or those of the family. Counselors may be required to attend family meetings to discuss progress or to explain therapy needs and requirements. It is extremely important for alcohol and drug abuse counselors to maintain patient confidentiality within the scope of the job.

Alcohol and drug abuse counselors work varied hours depending on their employment setting. Individuals are responsible to the supervisor of the department or the physician in charge.

Employment Opportunities

Alcohol and drug abuse counselors may work full- or part-time in a vast array of profit and not-for-profit employment settings including:

- Hospitals
- Schools
- Prisons
- Colleges and universities
- Private substance abuse centers
- Health maintenance organizations (HMO's)
- Self-employment
- Public substance abuse centers
- Mental health facilities
- Government agencies
- Social services organizations
- Corporate businesses

Expanding Opportunities for the Year 2000

The increase in drug and alcohol abuse will create a tremendous need for counselors. Individuals in the greatest demand will be those with the most education and training in substance abuse counseling.

Earnings

Alcohol and drug abuse counselors earn from $12,000 to $35,000 plus. Earnings depend on the specific em-

ployment setting and the size, prestige, and geographic location of the facility. Other factors include the experience and duties of the counselor.

Generally, the more education and experience, the higher the earnings will be. Counselors will also earn higher incomes in prestigious, private facilities.

Advancement Opportunities

Alcohol and drug abuse counselors can advance by obtaining experience and additional education to increase earnings and responsibilities. Counselors may also climb the career ladder by locating positions in prestigious facilities.

Many counselors advance to supervisory or administrative positions.

Education and Training

Education and training requirements for alcohol and drug abuse counselors vary from state to state and job to job. With more states starting to certify counselors, it is important for individuals to get a good education.

There are one-year certificate programs as well as two-year associate degrees, four-year bachelors' degrees and graduate degrees in alcohol and drug technology. Although some jobs just require a one-year certificate program, the minimum education recommended is an associate degree in alcohol and drug technology from an accredited college.

Experience and Qualifications

Certification requirements vary from state to state. Alcohol and drug abuse counselors may be certified by the National Association of Alcoholism and Drug Abuse Counselors (NAADAC) or be state-certified in certain states. In order to obtain certification, individuals must generally go through an accredited educational program, pass written and oral examinations, participate in supervised clinical experience, and have a taped sample of their clinical work.

For Additional Information: Individuals interested in pursuing careers in drug and alcohol counseling can obtain additional information by contacting the National Clearinghouse on Alcoholism and Drug Abuse Information (NCADI), Alcohol and Drug Problems Association (ADPA), the National Association of Alcoholism and Drug Abuse Counselors (NAADAC), National Association of Substance Abuse Trainers and Educators (NASATE), the National Institute on Alcohol Abuse and Alcoholism (NIAAA), the National Institute on Drug Abuse (NIDA), the American Association for Counseling and Development (AACD), the Council for Accreditation of Counseling and Related Education Programs (ACREP), the National Board for Certified Counselors (NBCC), and the National Academy of Certified Clinical Mental Health Counselors (NACCMHC).

TIPS

- You can obtain an entry-level or volunteer position in this field to obtain necessary experience.

- Job openings are often advertised in the newspaper classified section under "Alcohol and Drug Counselor," "Substance Abuse Counselor," "Mental Health Counseling," "Detox Clinics," "Health Care," etc.

- Colleges offering programs in alcohol and drug technology usually have a placement office that is aware of job openings in the field.

DIETITIAN

. . . .

Job Description: Design diets; analyze dietary needs; promote healthful eating habits; research nutritional needs and requirements.

Earnings: $15,000 to $45,000+

Recommended Education and Training: Minimum education is a bachelor's degree; some positions require a master's degree.

Skills and Personality Traits: Interpersonal skills; communication skills; computer capability; detail oriented; administrative skills; scientific aptitude.

Experience and Qualifications: Credentialing offered by the American Dietetic Association.

Job Description and Responsibilities

Dietitians are responsible for developing healthful diets by analyzing the nutritional needs of individuals.

In a clinical atmosphere, dietitians are responsible for handling, on a one-on-one basis, the nutritional needs of patients who are ill, injured, or infirm. Clinical dietitians or therapeutic dietitians, as they are sometimes called, work with patients in hospitals, nursing homes, extended care facilities, clinics, or doctors' offices in an attempt to develop nutritional plans.

Each patient is different. For example, a patient who has high blood pressure would not be on the same diet as a patient suffering from depression or diabetes. The dietitian will also be responsible for answering any questions patients may have, explaining all dietary allowances and restrictions, and coordinating dietary prescriptions with the menus planned by the facility.

In other situations, the dietitian will be required to advise, counsel, and educate individuals on how to stay healthy and prevent disease. Dietitians who handle these types of functions are called community dietitians. They work in clinics, home health agencies, and human service organizations. In this capacity, dietitians evaluate the eating habits of individuals or families and develop an economical nutrition plan for them to follow. They may educate individuals or groups on the nutritional analysis of foods and explain what type of foods are high in saturated fats or what foods are high in fiber. Disease prevention through nutrition is an important function for community dietitians.

Depending on their specific situation, some dietitians analyze the nutritional content of specific foods or combinations of foods. Others prepare literature on the nutritional analysis of foods, dietary needs, and healthful diets.

Dietitians working in large facilities may be called management dietitians. These individuals work in hospitals, health care facilities, prisons, schools, corporate cafeterias, and other large facilities. Management dietitians are responsible for planning all the meals in these facilities for patients, employees, and visitors.

Another area of specialization for dietitians is research. Research is conducted in a number of areas from nutritional analysis of foods to nutritional requirements of individuals with certain diseases. More companies are attempting to develop new products that are nutritionally sound and lower in calories and fat. Individuals working in this field may work in corporate food research labs, medical centers, and educational institutions.

Employment Opportunities

Dietitians may specialize in research or clinical and community nutrition, or may be management dietitians responsible for the planning and preparation of meals for large facilities. Dietitians work in a vast array of settings including:

- Hospitals
- Nursing homes
- Food service companies
- Prisons
- Schools

- Corporate cafeterias
- Community health programs
- Clinics
- Consulting
- Private practice
- Hotel and restaurant chains
- Extended care facilities
- Corporations (research)
- Health maintenance organizations

Expanding Opportunities for the Year 2000

With the current knowledge of the correlation between food, nutrition, and disease risk, clinical dietitians who specialize in obesity, kidney disease, heart disease, diabetes, and cancer will be in demand.

Earnings

Full-time dietitians earn from $15,000 to $45,000 or more. Factors affecting earnings include the specific type of facility and its size, prestige, and geographic location. Other factors include the responsibilities, experience, and education level of the dietitian.

The average salary for dietitians is around $30,000. Individuals with postgraduate education, experience, and a great deal of responsibility will earn salaries at the higher end of the scale. Those doing research for large corporations will also earn higher salaries than individuals working for hospitals, schools, and public programs.

Advancement Opportunities

Dietitians can follow a number of paths to career advancement depending on the direction that they want to pursue. Individuals can locate similar positions in larger or more prestigious facilities, resulting in increased responsibilities and earnings. They might also choose specialization as their path to advancement. Clinical dieticians may, for example, specialize in fields including obesity, kidney disease, heart disease, diabetes, or cancer. Other fields of specialization include nutrition for pediatrics, critical care patients, or gerontology.

Dietitians may climb the career ladder by becoming supervisors or managers of a dietary department.

Education and Training

Dietitians should have a minimum of a bachelor's degree in foods, nutrition, or food service administration. Individuals interested in becoming registered dietitians should complete their education at a college or university accredited by the American Dietetic Association. Courses for dietitians include nutrition, chemistry, microbiology, physiology, math, statistics, psychology, sociology, economics, biology, and computer science and technology.

Some positions may require a postgraduate degree. These include research, teaching, and public health positions. As a rule, the more education, the more options that will be open to the individual, both in attaining a job and in career advancement.

Experience and Qualifications

Many employers prefer that their dietitians be professionally credentialed and registered. In order to obtain these credentials, individuals must fulfill the requirements of the American Dietetic Association. These include completion of a bachelor's degree in foods and nutrition or institution management from an accredited program, plus clinical experience. Clinical experience

may be obtained by attending one of the accredited four-year university or college programs that combine both the academic requirements and the clinical experience. It can also be obtained by fulfilling a 900-hour accredited internship program or an approved preprofessional practice program. One of the reasons many people, especially career changers, opt for the preprofessional practice program is that it can be undertaken on a part-time basis.

For Additional Information: Career-related literature can be obtained from the American Dietetic Association (ADA). Additional information regarding specific careers in this field is available from the US Office of Personnel Management and the Veterans Administration (VA).

TIPS

- Obtain the best education possible. More options will be open to those with postgraduate degrees. If you can't attend graduate school full time, take courses on a part-time basis while working.

- With the current interest in health and fitness, you may be able to find a part-time job as a consultant for a health club or diet center.

- Job openings may be advertised in the newspaper display or classified section under "Dietitian," "Nutritionist," "Health Care," "Community Health," "Public Health," "School Dietitian," etc.

- The federal government often has openings for dietitians. Contact either the Veterans Administration or the United States Office of Personnel Management to obtain requirements and information.

EEG TECHNOLOGIST/TECHNICIAN

Job Description: Operate and maintain electroencephalographs; read and interpret EEG tapes.

Earnings: $15,000 to $33,000

Recommended Education and Training: High school diploma; on-the-job training or formal training.

Skills and Personality Traits: Manual dexterity; personable; good eyesight; communication skills; electronic aptitude.

Experience and Qualifications: Many jobs do not require experience; credentialing is available.

Job Description and Responsibilities

EEG stands for electroencephalogram. These are records of brain waves that are important in treating and diagnosing many medical conditions.

EEG's are taken with an instrument called an electroencephalograph. These units are used as diagnostic tools to diagnose the amount of injury patients have sustained from strokes, brain tumors, metabolic disorders, epilepsy, etc. EEG's are also used to monitor patients in surgery, to determine causes of behavioral problems, and to measure the effects of diseases on the brain. The EEG tests not only brain waves, but heart activity too.

EEG technologists and technicians are responsible for operating electroenccphalographs. Generally, individuals who are credentialed in this area are referred to as technologists while those who are not are called technicians.

EEG techs have a variety of duties depending on the specific job and their training. The first thing that must be done is to make sure that all equipment is working properly. Next, individuals are responsible for taking a patient's medical history and putting patients at ease.

EEG techs apply electrodes to various spots on the patient's body and head before performing the procedure. The procedure may be performed while the patient is resting, sleeping, or moving about in normal everyday activities. Various stimuli may also be added to determine reactions.

The information recorded from the EEG will be documented on a paper tape and may look very much like a map or chart. After the procedure is completed, the EEG technologist or technician may be responsible for reviewing and reading the paper tape and determining what sections should be shown to the patient's doctor.

The greater the responsibilities of the individual, the more training will be required. For example, EEG technologists working in operating rooms must be thoroughly familiar with anesthesia's effect on brain waves. Those working in other areas must be versed in other technologies. Throughout every procedure, the EEG technologist or technician must be aware when a major change is occurring so that a physician can be alerted.

Individuals will be responsible to either the physician or the supervisor of the EEG laboratory depending on the specific situation.

Employment Opportunities

EEG technologists and technicians are usually employed full-time in hospitals. However, individuals may work in a variety of other settings including:

- Neurology laboratories
- Neurologists' offices

- Neurosurgeons' offices
- Group medical practices
- Health maintenance organizations (HMO's)
- Urgent care centers
- Emergency clinics
- Psychiatric facilities

Expanding Opportunities for the Year 2000

There is a continuing trend for neurologists, group practices, and health maintenance organizations (HMO's) to have their own equipment for these types of tests. While jobs will be plentiful for EEG technologists and technicians in hospitals, there will also be a tremendous need for individuals in this field in outpatient settings.

Earnings

Earnings for EEG technologists and technicians range from approximately $15,000 to $33,000 per year. Salaries depend on the geographic area that the individual is employed in as well as the specific type, size, and prestige of the facility. Other factors include experience, responsibilities, and qualifications.

Those who have experience, are registered, and are working in larger metropolitan cities will be compensated at the high end of the scale.

EEG technologists and technicians usually have their salaries augmented by benefit packages.

Advancement Opportunities

With experience, an EEG technologist may advance to supervisory positions including Chief EEG Technologist, Special Procedures Instructor, or Training Program Director. These jobs would result in increased earnings and responsibility.

Education and Training

Aspiring EEG technologists or technicians can take two paths regarding education and training. One method is to receive on-the-job training. The other is to take a formal training program in EEG technology.

Formal programs are offered in many community colleges, colleges, universities, vocational or technical schools, hospitals, and medical centers. Depending on the specific program, completion may take from one to two years. The Joint Review Committee for the Accreditation of EEG Technology Training Programs approves some but not all programs.

Students in formal training programs will receive classroom instruction and laboratory experience. Individuals completing this training will be awarded either an associate degree or a certificate.

Experience and Qualifications

Many positions in this field are entry level and will not require any special prior experience.

Although it is not usually necessary for those just entering the field, credentialing may be needed for advancement. Individuals may become credentialed through the American Board of Registration of Electroencephalographic Technologists and receive the title of Registered EEG Technologist.

For Additional Information: Individuals interested in a career in EEG technology can obtain additional information by contacting the American Society of Electroneurodiagnostic Technologists (ASET), the Joint Review Committee for the Accreditation of EEG Technology Training Programs, the American Board of Registration for Electroencephalographic Technologists (ABRET), or their local hospital.

TIPS

- Most of the formal programs in this field offer placement services.

- Job openings may be advertised in the newspaper's classified section under headings such as "Health Care," "EEG Technologist," "EEG Technician," or "Technology."

- Contact personnel offices of hospital and health care facilities to inquire about job openings or training programs.

EKG TECHNICIAN

Job Description: Operate electrocardiograph; interpret graphs; write reports.

Earnings: $13,000 to $26,000

Recommended Education and Training: High school diploma; on-the-job training.

Skills and Personality Traits: Mechanically inclined; personable; familiarity with medical terminology; communication skills.

Experience and Qualifications: Experience in the health care field helpful; voluntary credentialing available.

Job Description and Responsibilities

Electrocardiographs are machines that record graphic tracings of heartbeats called electrocardiograms. Electrocardiograms are referred to as EKG's. They are used for a variety of reasons including diagnosis and treatment of heart and circulatory problems.

EKG technicians operate electrocardiograph machines. Responsibilities of EKG technicians will vary depending on experience and training.

After making sure that the EKG machine is working correctly, the individual will try to put the patient at ease and explain the procedure. The individual will then apply a type of cream to the patient's skin and attach electrodes to the correct spots on the chest, arms, and legs. The individual must be sure to place the electrodes in the correct places or the readings will not be accurate. When the machine is turned on it will record the action and reactions of the heart. The technician must have the ability to recognize problems that are caused by technical errors including crossed leads or electrical interference.

After the procedure is completed, the technician will remove the electrodes and prepare the EKG for the physician. Most often it is computers that analyze the tracings, but the technician may be required to enter the correct information into the computer. The individual may also be required to go over the tracings to see if there are any major deviations from the norm.

EKG technicians may work various shifts depending on the specific job. They are responsible to the physician in charge or the EKG laboratory supervisor.

Employment Opportunities

EKG technicians can work full time or may find part-time employment. The majority of EKG technicians in the country work in hospital settings. With the advances in cardiology medicine, however, there are opportunities in other settings including:

- Medical centers
- Cardiologists' offices
- Cardiac rehabilitation centers
- Health maintenance organizations (HMO's)
- Health clinics
- Long-term care facilities
- Nursing homes

Expanding Opportunities for the Year 2000

Because heart disease is a major problem in this country, new diagnostic procedures are constantly being developed. EKG technicians who continue their training will be the most marketable. Without additional training, however, individuals will only have the ability to do basic tests.

Earnings

Annual earnings for full-time EKG technicians can range from approximately $13,000 to $26,000. Variables affecting salaries include the experience level and responsibilities of the individual as well as the specific facility and geographical location.

Those who have attained some experience will be compensated towards the middle of the scale while those who perform more sophisticated or complicated tests will have earnings at the high end of the pay scale. Earnings are also generally higher for individuals working in facilities in large, metropolitan cities.

Many EKG technicians have their salaries augmented by liberal fringe benefit packages.

Advancement Opportunities

EKG technicians can advance by moving into supervisory or administrative positions within the department.

EKG technicians who acquire additional training and skills have the best chance of career advancement. With the proper training, individuals can move into specialized positions. Some EKG technicians who obtain extensive training may also climb the career ladder by becoming invasive or noninvasive cardiology technologists.

Education and Training

EKG technicians should be high school graduates. Courses in the sciences, including biology, health, and human anatomy, will be useful.

EKG technicians receive on-the-job training by working either with a cardiologist or an EKG supervisor. The basic training is approximately a month to six weeks in duration and will prepare the EKG technician for basic EKG procedures. Another five months of training will prepare the EKG technician for other tasks such as handling ill patients, interpreting graphs, and writing reports for doctors to review.

Individuals performing specialized EKG tests such as ambulatory monitoring and stress tests must have four more months of training.

Experience and Qualifications

While some facilities prefer to train individuals who have some familiarity with the health care field, there are generally no experience requirements. An eagerness to learn the field will qualify most individuals for in-house, on-the-job training.

EKG technicians do not have to be licensed and credentialing is voluntary. Credentialing can be obtained through the Cardiovascular Credentialing International and National Board of Cardiovascular Testing. Credentialing shows professional competence and may give one applicant an edge over another.

For Additional Information: For more information contact the National Society of Cardiovascular Technology/National Society of Pulmonary Technology (NSCT/NSPT) and the Cardiovascular Credentialing International and National Board of Cardiovascular Testing (CCI/NBCT).

TIPS

• If you are still in school, you may consider either volunteering or getting a part-time or summer job working in a health care setting.

• Many health care facilities, vocational technical schools, high schools, and community colleges sponsor health career days where interested individuals can learn more about careers in these fields.

• Consider sending your resume with a short cover letter to the personnel directors of health care facilities. Remember to request that your resume be kept on file for the future if there are no current openings.

• Jobs may be advertised in the classified section of local newspapers under headings such as "EKG Technician," "Health Care," "Physician's Office," "Hospitals," "Cardiac Rehabilitation Center," "Health Maintenance Organization," etc.

EMERGENCY MEDICAL TECHNICIAN

Job Description: Provide emergency medical treatment; assess and monitor patient's condition; drive ambulances or vans.

Earnings: $15,000 to $36,000+

Recommended Education and Training: High school diploma; standard training course in emergency medical care.

Skills and Personality Traits: Emotional stability; enjoy helping others; good judgment; physical stamina; ability to work under stress.

Experience and Qualifications: A valid driver's license required; certification/registration available.

Job Description and Responsibilities

Emergency medical technicians provide emergency medical help. EMT's may be called in to deal with accident victims, heart attacks, stab or gunshot wounds, drug overdoses, poisonings, etc. While EMT's are not doctors, they are highly trained in emergency lifesaving techniques.

There are a number of levels of emergency medical technicians. The entry-level job may be referred to as EMT-Ambulance, EMT-A, or basic EMT. Other levels are EMT-Intermediate, EMT-Paramedic, and EMT-Defibrillator.

Levels of the job are based on the amount of training the individual has received and will affect the procedures they can perform. For example, in most states EMT-Intermediates are allowed to treat trauma patients with intravenous fluids, anti-shock garments, and airway management techniques. EMT-Ambulance personnel are usually not permitted to provide these additional services.

EMT-Paramedics are trained in advanced life support skills. These individuals often work under the direction of a physician using radio communication and administering oral or intravenous drugs, performing endotracheal intubation, and interpreting EKGs. Some EMT-Paramedics may also use defibrillators when required.

EMT-Defibrillators are trained in administering electrical defibrillation, which can be used to resuscitate some heart attack victims. This level of EMT is a relatively new designation. It was designed to provide EMT-Ambulance people with additional training required to administer these procedures.

Once an EMT team arrives at the scene, their first responsibility is to assess the situation. They may work with other emergency departments including police and firefighters to determine priorities for handling the situation.

Once priority decisions are made, EMT's are responsible for providing the appropriate emergency care. Individuals may handle procedures that they have been trained to do or may be in radio contact with medical staff who can give them step-by-step instructions. Depending on the situation, the EMT may perform CPR, treat patients for shock, resuscitate heart attack patients, control bleeding, open airways, assist in the birth of a baby, or handle a vast array of other procedures.

The EMT will transmit information to the dispatcher or hospital regarding the type and extent of emergencies. Individuals may give patient's vital signs, symptoms, and condition. EMT's may be directed to the closest hospital with the appropriate equipment or to a specialty facility depending on the situation.

After placing a patient in the care of a facility, the EMT must make sure that the ambulance is ready for the next call. Linens, blankets, and bandages may need replacing, and equipment may need to be sterilized.

Other functions of the EMT may include writing reports on patients transported, checking to be sure that the ambulance is in good working order, and supplying the vehicle with the needed equipment.

Working hours will vary for EMT's depending on the specific shift. This is a difficult, challenging, and rewarding job. Most people who are performing this service are saving lives on a daily basis.

Employment Opportunities

Emergency medical technicians can work for:

- Hospitals
- Medical centers
- Fire departments
- Police departments
- Rescue squad departments
- Private ambulance companies

Expanding Opportunities for the Year 2000

Financial difficulties are causing many not-for-profit hospitals, municipal police, and fire and rescue squads to cut back on staff and services. These organizations must then contract with private ambulance companies to perform emergency services.

It is also important to note that highly trained EMT's will be extremely marketable in the future.

Earnings

Earnings for emergency medical technicians vary depending on the specific type of work setting and geographic location, as well as training and experience.

Annual earnings can range from $15,000 to $36,000 or more. Salaries are to a great extent based on the training and level of EMT the individual achieves.

EMT's working for fire departments will usually earn more than those performing similar duties in hospitals or for private ambulance services. Highest salaries will go to paramedics with experience working in large, metropolitan cities.

Advancement Opportunities

Emergency medical technicians can advance by seeking additional training, learning more skills, and obtaining experience. They can move from an EMT-Ambulance to an EMT-Intermediate and up to an EMT-Paramedic.

Education and Training

EMT personnel must hold a high school diploma or equivalent. They must also complete training in emergency medical care techniques. The basic standard training course is offered nationwide by police and fire departments, ambulance corps, health departments, hospitals, medical centers, colleges, universities, and medical schools. The first phase of the nondegree course lasts approximately 110 hours and covers instruction and practice in emergencies and basic life support techniques. It is the training required to become an EMT-Ambulance.

Additional training includes a two-day class in the removal of trapped victims and a five-day course on driving ambulances and other emergency vehicles. Individuals interested in training for the EMT-Defibrillation level must complete an intensive course on defibrillation.

Training for the EMT-Intermediate level includes the basic EMT training as well as some of the EMT-Paramedic course material. Specific training requirements vary from state to state.

Those interested in becoming EMT-Paramedics must go through a program which usually lasts about nine months. Programs are accredited by the American Medical Association's Committee on Allied Health Education and Accreditation.

Experience and Qualifications

Qualifications vary for emergency medical technicians. As a rule, individuals must be at least 18 years old and hold a valid driver's license.

Emergency medical technicians may be certified by either the specific state's certifying agency or the National Registry of Emergency Medical Technicians. While this is not always a requirement, it is certainly recommended.

To earn the title of Registered EMT-Ambulance, individuals must graduate from an approved EMT training program. They must also obtain a certain degree of experience and pass both a written and practical examination administered by either the National Registry of Emergency Medical Technicians or the specific state's certifying agency. In order to keep this certification, individuals must be employed in the field, continue their education, and pay a fee at regular timed intervals.

Those interested in being registered as EMT-Intermediates must be registered EMT-A's, pass an examination, take 35 to 55 more hours of classroom study, obtain a certain amount of clinical experience, and go through a field internship.

Requirements for EMT-Paramedics include current registration or state certification as an EMT-Ambulance, completion of the EMT-Paramedic training program, six months of field experience, and taking and passing both a written and practical examination.

For Additional Information: For more information contact the National Registry of Emergency Medical Technicians (NREMT), the National Association of Emergency Medical Technicians (NAEMT), or the Emergency Medical Service Director in your particular state.

TIPS

- A good way to make sure this is the career for you is volunteering to work on your local ambulance corps.

- Job openings may be advertised in the newspaper classified section under heading classifications such as "Emergency Medical Technicians," "EMT's," "Emergency Medical Service," "Ambulance Technicians," "Rescue Squad," "Health Care," etc.

- Send your resume and a short cover letter to medical centers; hospitals; private ambulance companies; and municipal fire, police, and rescue squads. Request that your resume be kept on file if there are no current openings.

- If you are or were a medic in the armed forces, you already have valuable experience in this field.

MEDICAL RECORDS TECHNICIAN

Job Description: Assemble and organize medical records; code procedures and diagnoses, tabulate data.

Earnings: $15,000 to $25,000

Recommended Education and Training: Associate degree from an accredited program in medical records technology.

Skills and Personality Traits: Reliabilty; fastidiousness; computer capability; good communication skills.

Experience and Qualifications: Knowledge of medical terms.

Job Description and Responsibilities

Hospitals and other facilities dealing in health care must maintain a vast number of medical records. These records include patients' medical history, symptoms, test results, diagnoses, medications, admission dates, discharge dates, names of attending physicians, and physician notes.

Medical records technicians handle the organization and assembly of these medical records. They work with others in the medical records department to establish files for every patient who visits the facility. It is extremely important to health care facilities to handle this in an accurate and timely manner in order to be reimbursed properly and adequately.

Medical records technicians may also be responsible for tabulating and analyzing data. This information could be used for many purposes. It may, for example, be used to check quality assurance or to determine the plausibility of adding a new type of health unit to the facility.

Medical records technicians may have supervisory responsibilities over clerks working in the department. They are responsible to the medical records supervisor.

Employment Opportunities

With the great demand for qualified people in this profession, there is often flexibility in working hours. Medical records technicians may find full or part-time employment in a variety of settings such as:

- Hospitals
- Nursing homes
- Health maintenance organizations (HMO's)
- Private or public health clinics
- Physicians' offices
- Home health agencies

Expanding Opportunities for the Year 2000

With the rise in health care costs, hospitals will be in great need of accurate medical records in order to obtain government, health care agency, and insurance reimbursement. Providing this accurate information is the job of medical records technicians.

Earnings

Annual earnings for medical records technicians range from approximately $15,000 to $25,000. Those who have supervisory positions will earn more. Factors af-

fecting salary include the individual's experience and responsibilities. Other factors include the specific facility and its size, prestige, and geographic location. Individuals working in health care facilities will usually have their earnings augmented by benefit packages.

Advancement Opportunities

Medical records technicians can advance by specializing in a particular area of medical records technology.

Some climb the career ladder by teaching. This method of advancement will usually require a master's degree in either health administration or education. Others become supervisors or managers of either the entire medical records department or a specific area within the department.

Education and Training

There are two ways of obtaining the training necessary to become a credentialed medical records technician. One is to complete a two-year course and obtain an associate degree from a college offering an accredited program in medical records technology. The other is to graduate from an independent study program offered by the American Medical Record Association. In order to participate in independent study, an individual must have 30 hours of credit in areas prescribed by the AMRA.

Once the educational requirements are met, medical records technicians may become credentialed by passing a written examination sponsored by the American Medical Record Association. While credentials are not mandatory, most employers prefer that technicians have them.

Experience and Qualifications

Medical records technicians should have a complete knowledge and understanding of medical terminology and procedures.

For Additional Information: Individuals interested in learning more about careers in medical records technology should contact the American Medical Record Association (AMRA).

TIPS

• Once you obtain basic experience working as a medical records technician, try to learn extra skills so that you can specialize. This will help you advance and increase your income.

• Take computer courses or workshops. This will put you a step above others who do not have this skill.

• If you are still in school, work summers or part-time in a health care facility as a medical records clerk. This will give you hands-on experience.

PHYSICIAN ASSISTANT (PA)
· ·

Job Description: Take medical histories; examine patients; order lab tests; treat minor medical problems.

Earnings: $24,000 to $40,000

Recommended Education and Training: Degree from an accredited P.A. program.

Skills and Personality Traits: Caring; compassion; emotional stability; dependability.

Experience and Qualifications: State certification exam may be required.

Job Description and Responsibilities

Physician assistants work under the supervision of licensed physicians. Their responsibilities may be determined by either a supervising physician or the state's regulatory agency. In some states, therefore, individuals will be able to perform duties which cannot be carried out by physician assistants in other states.

The services of a physician assistant free up the physician's time to handle other important functions. In many situations, physicians are not always available and the assistant can provide necessary services. The physician assistant may work with the doctor when available or on a telephone to consult when there is no physician at the scene.

Physician assistants may be responsible for treating minor medical emergencies including cuts, bruises, abrasions, and burns. They may also handle both preoperative and postoperative patient care. Those who have the training may work in operating rooms. Others are responsible for taking patient medical histories and performing physical examinations. Some physician assistants do the examinations required by insurance companies for college-bound students.

Physician assistants may also examine patients who are ill. Sometimes PA's are required to make a preliminary diagnosis of a patient's illness and in doing so may order laboratory tests. Depending on the state, some physician assistants prescribe treatments and recommend medication and drug therapies.

PA's may work in general medicine in private practice offices, hospitals, and clinics or in specialty areas. They may work under physicians who specialize in family medicine, pediatrics, internal medicine, general surgery, emergency medicine, or many other areas.

PA's work a variety of hours depending on their employment situation. They are responsible to the physician they work with.

Employment Opportunities

PA's work in most of the same settings as physicians. These include:

- Physicians' offices
- Medical groups
- Hospitals
- Health maintenance organizations (HMO's)
- Public health clinics
- Prisons
- Nursing homes
- Extended care facilities
- Rehabilitation centers
- Facilities for the disabled
- Facilities for the mentally retarded
- Schools, colleges, universities

Expanding Opportunities for the Year 2000

Currently, most physician assistants work in private medical practices and hospitals. However, trends indicate there will be a growing demand for these professionals in a variety of other facilities that use the services of physicians. These include nursing homes, public health clinics, and health maintenance organizations (HMO's).

Earnings

Physician assistants have earnings ranging from $24,000 to $40,000, depending on the individual's experience, responsibilities, qualifications, and training.

Other factors affecting earnings include the specific facility the individual is working in and its size, prestige, and geographic location. Most physician assistants' earnings range from $29,000 to $35,000. PA's with more experience working in large metropolitan cities will move to the top of the pay scale faster.

Advancement Opportunities

After obtaining experience, physician assistants can advance into positions in larger or more prestigious settings.

Other physician assistants climb the career ladder by getting additional education so that they can specialize in fields such as emergency medicine, surgery, or neonatology.

Education and Training

Recommended educational requirements for physician assistants include graduation from an accredited program. Accredited PA programs lead to a certificate, an associate degree, a bachelor's degree, or a master's degree.

Physician assistant programs are usually two years in duration and include classroom instruction and clinical experience. Subjects cover human anatomy, physiology, microbiology, biochemistry, nutrition, clinical pharmacology, clinical medicine, geriatric and home health care, medical ethics, and disease prevention.

The clinical experience portion of the program covers areas including family medicine, general surgery, inpatient and ambulatory medicine, obstetrics and gynecology, geriatrics, emergency medicine, internal medicine, pediatrics, and ambulatory psychiatry.

Postgraduate residencies are available in a number of specialties.

Experience and Qualifications

Qualifications for physician assistants depend on the state they work in. Some states require individuals to pass a certifying exam in addition to completing an accredited educational program.

For Additional Information: Individuals interested in learning more about careers as physician assistants can obtain additional information by contacting the American Academy of Physician Assistants (AAPA), the Association of Physician Assistant Programs

(APAP), and the National Commission on Certification of Physician Assistants, Inc. (NCCPA).

TIPS

- Prior experience working in the health care field is a plus for getting into an accredited program.

- Even if physicians are not advertising for physician assistants, it does not mean they would not consider hiring one. Send your resume and a short cover letter to physicians' offices, hospitals, health care facilities, and clinics.

- Part-time work or flexible scheduling is often available for physician assistants.

CLINICAL LABORATORY TECHNOLOGIST
. . . .

Job Description: Perform laboratory tests; examine blood, tissue, and other body substances; make cultures of body fluid and tissue samples; type and cross-match blood samples.

Earnings: $18,000 to $34,000+

Recommended Education and Training: Bachelor's degree in medical technology or life sciences.

Skills and Personality Traits: Manual dexterity; normal vision; communication skills; ability to work under pressure; computer skills; analytical skills.

Experience and Qualifications: State licensing; credentialing required for some jobs.

Job Description and Responsibilities

Clinical laboratory technologists perform a variety of medical tests on patients. These may include chemical, biological, hematological, microscopic, immunologic, and bacteriological laboratory tests. Technologists use microscopes, chemical analyzers, and computers to perform these tests and analyze the results.

All tests must be ordered by a physician and may be used for a variety of reasons. They may indicate diseases or infections. They might also detect specific illnesses, help with diagnosis and treatment, or be used to determine the status of an individual's health.

Lab technologists' responsibilities and duties depend on the specific job, the employment setting, and the individual's education and experience.

Technologists draw blood and collect samples of tissues or other body substances to be analyzed and examined. In some situations, technologists take specimens and make cultures in order to analyze them. They may examine the cultures with a microscope, looking for parasites, microorganisms, fungi, or other bacteria.

Clinical lab technologists might be required to analyze samples for chemical content. For example, they might prepare slides with body tissue, blood, or fluid to determine abnormalities such as cancer cells. Another duty of the clinical lab technologist includes typing and cross-matching blood samples for transfusions.

Individuals may specialize in clinical laboratory testing. Those who prepare slides of body cells and examine them for abnormalities are called cytotechnologists. Clinical chemistry technologists prepare specimens and analyze the chemical and hormonal content of body fluids. Microbiology technologists examine and identify bacteria and other microorganisms. Blood bank technologists collect, type, and prepare blood for transfusions. Immunology technologists examine elements and responses of the immune system to foreign substances.

Clinical laboratory technologists work various hours depending on their shift. Individuals are responsible to the chief medical technologist, the laboratory manager, or the physician in charge.

Employment Opportunities

Employment possibilities include:

- Hospitals
- Physicians' offices
- Medical centers
- Group medical practices
- Independent laboratories
- Clinics
- Health maintenance organizations (HMO's)
- Pharmaceutical companies
- Public health agencies
- Research institutes
- Extended care facilities
- Urgi-centers
- Surgi-centers
- Commercial laboratories

Expanding Opportunities for the Year 2000

There will be a great demand for lab technologists as a result of innovative technology leading to newer and more powerful diagnostic tests.

Laboratory technologists will also find new opportunities in research labs working to find treatments and cures for cancer, AIDS, and other deadly diseases.

With an increase in home medical tests, pharmaceutical companies will require a greater number of laboratory technologists to develop products.

Earnings

Earnings for clinical laboratory technologists range from approximately $18,000 to $34,000 or more. Factors affecting earnings include the specific employment situation and geographic location as well as the responsibilities, experience, and training of individuals.

Technologists just starting out will have earnings ranging from $18,000 to $23,000. Those with more experience and responsibilities earn between $23,000 and $34,000 plus. Individuals working in larger, metropolitan cities will earn more than their counterparts in less urban areas.

Advancement Opportunities

Clinical laboratory technologists can advance their careers in a number of ways including additional experience and education. Some individuals locate similar positions in larger or more prestigious facilities. Technologists might also land supervisory positions or administrative jobs such as laboratory manager or chief medical technologist.

Education and Training

It is recommended that clinical laboratory technologists have a bachelor's degree with a major in either medical technology or one of the life sciences.

Many colleges and universities, as well as a number of hospitals affiliated with colleges or universities, offer majors in medical technology. It is important that the college, university, or hospital be accredited by the Committee on Allied Health Education and Accreditation, in cooperation with the National Accrediting Agency for Clinical Laboratory Sciences.

The programs in medical technology consist of classroom and lab work in chemistry, microbiology, biological sciences, math, computers, management, business, and clinical laboratory skills.

Graduate programs in medical technology and clinical laboratory sciences are also available.

Experience and Qualifications

Clinical laboratory technologists may be required to be state-licensed, depending on the state in which they are working.

Certification is required for certain positions. Individuals may receive certification from a number of organizations including the Board of Registry of the American Society of Clinical Pathologists in conjunction with the American Association of Blood Banks, the American Medical Technologists, the National Certification Agency for Medical Laboratory Personnel, and the Credentialing Commission of the International Society for Clinical Laboratory Technology. Requirements for certification vary with the specific organization.

For Additional Information: There are a number of organizations individuals can contact for more information about careers in clinical laboratory technology. These include the American Society of Clinical Pathologists (ASCP), American Medical Technologists (AMT), American Association for Clinical Chemistry (AACC), the American Association of Blood Banks (AABB), the American Society of Cytology (ASC), the National Certification Agency for Medical Laboratory Personnel (NCAMLP), the International Society for Clinical Laboratory Technology (ISCLT), the Committee on Allied Health Education and Accreditation (CAHEA), and the National Institutes of Health (NIH).

TIPS

- Opportunities for clinical laboratory technologists are often available in Veterans Administration Medical Centers.

- Federal jobs may be available with the National Institutes of Health.

- Job openings may be advertised in the newspaper's classified section under headings such as "Health Care," "Hospitals," "Laboratories," "Clinical Laboratory Technologists," "Lab Technologists," etc.

- Send your resume with a short cover letter to the personnel directors of hospitals, physician's offices, medical centers, independent laboratories, etc. Request that your resume be kept on file if there are no current openings.

- Colleges and universities offering degree programs in medical technology usually have placement services for their graduates.

HEALTH SERVICES ADMINISTRATOR

Job Description: Overall management of health care institution; assess the need for services; hire personnel; supervise assistant administrators.

Earnings: $35,000 to $150,000+

Recommended Education and Training: Master's degree in health services administration, hospital administration, or business administration.

Skills and Personality Traits: Leadership ability; managerial skills; communication skills; ability to deal with press and media.

Experience and Qualifications: Experience necessary; state licensing required for administrators of nursing homes and extended care facilities.

Job Description and Responsibilities

Health services administrators are responsible for overseeing the operation and management of health care facilities. Specific duties and responsibilities vary depending on the size of the facility.

In smaller facilities or agencies, administrators are responsible for the overall direction and financial management of the institution or agency. Administrators in these situations may also be called the CEO or chief executive officer.

In larger facilities, the CEO may delegate duties to other administrators. For example, financial management will be delegated to a chief fiscal officer; personnel requirements to a personnel director, planning to a planning officer; public relations and marketing to a P.R. director; and supervision of various other patient services and ancillary departments to associate or deputy administrators.

The top health services administrator is expected to supervise all assistant and deputy administrators. Day-to-day decisions are also handled by assistant and deputy administrators or directors who are assigned projects within the scope of their job.

Depending on the type of facility, administrators may have a great deal of direct contact with patients or this contact may be limited. For example, administrators of nursing homes or extended care facilities will usually have more patient contact than their counterparts working in hospitals.

There is a great deal of responsibility in this type of job. For instance, administrators must prepare for periodic inspections by government agencies, insurance companies, and third-party reimbursers. These visits are extremely important to health care facilities. A negative report can mean fines, loss of public confidence, or the loss of revenue.

Health services administrators work long hours, often under tremendous pressure and in stressful situations. As all operational occurrences in the facility fall into their area of responsibility, they are always on call.

Employment Opportunities

Health services administrators may work as chief or executive administrators, assistants to the administrator, assistant administrators, or associate administrators. They work in a variety of health care settings including:

- Hospitals
- Nursing homes
- Extended care facilities
- Health maintenance organizations (HMO's)
- Urgi-centers
- Surgi-centers

- Rehabilitation facilities
- Psychiatric facilities
- Large medical groups

Expanding Opportunities for the Year 2000

Due to the growing population of older Americans, the demand for more facilities dealing with both the aging population and long-term care is expected to increase significantly.

In addition, the anticipated availability of some type of universal health insurance will create unprecedented access to health care for those currently uninsured or under-insured.

Earnings

Earnings of health services administrators can vary tremendously depending on a number of factors. These include the specific facility or agency, size, prestige, location, and type of ownership. Other factors are responsibilities, duties, education, and experience.

Annual earnings for health services administrators can range from $35,000 to $150,000 or more. Individuals with limited experience working in small facilities or agencies will earn salaries ranging from $35,000 to $50,000. Those working in larger facilities will have earnings from $45,000 to $70,000. Health services administrators with a great deal of experience and responsibility, working in very large facilities or multi-hospital systems, can earn from $70,000 to $150,000 plus.

In addition to salaries, most health services administrators receive liberal benefit packages to augment their earnings.

Advancement Opportunities

Health services administrators can advance their careers in a number of ways. Assistants to the director or administrator may become the assistant director or associate director.

Health services administrators can also progress by locating similar positions in larger, more complex facilities. This will result in increased responsibilities and earnings.

Education and Training

Health services administrators are usually required to have a master's degree in hospital administration, public health, or health administration. Master's degree programs in these areas are two to three years in duration and often include supervised administrative experience.

In order to be admitted to graduate school, individuals must have their bachelor's degree. Undergraduate majors may be in areas of business administration, health administration, liberal arts, and social sciences.

Experience and Qualifications

Health services administrators gain experience through internships, in jobs as department heads, or in other managerial capacities.

State licensing is necessary for health service administrators working in nursing homes and long-term care facilities. In order to obtain a state license, individuals must complete a state-approved training program, continue their education, and pass a licensing examination. Some states also have additional requirements.

For Additional Information: Individuals interested in learning more about health care facility administration can obtain additional information from the American College of Healthcare Executives (ACHE), the Association of University Programs in Health Administration (AUPHA), the American College of Health Care Administrators (ACHCA), and the American Association of Homes for the Aging (AAHA).

TIPS

• Colleges and universities offering degrees in this field usually have job placement services.

• Many cities host employment agencies specializing in careers in health care.

• Job openings are often advertised in the classified sections of newspapers. Look under "Health Care," "Long Term Care," "Facility Management," "Health Services Administrator," "Nursing Homes," "Health Care Management," and "Health Care Administration."

DISPENSING OPTICIAN

Job Description: Fill eyeglass prescriptions; assist customers in choosing frames; adjust finished glasses.

Earnings: $15,000 to $35,000

Recommended Education and Training: Apprenticeship; associate degree in ophthalmic dispensing.

Skills and Personality Traits: Manual dexterity; math and science skills; communication skills.

Experience and Qualifications: State licensing.

Job Description and Responsibilities

The primary function of a dispensing optician is to prepare eyeglass or lens prescriptions provided by either optometrists or ophthalmologists.

Corrective lenses are made by grinding down special lens glass in a specific, measured, scientific manner. The prescription will tell a technician exactly how to prepare the lenses. Each prescription performs a different function. The goal is for the individual to see better by correcting the dysfunction with the prepared glasses.

When a customer comes into an optical store, the optician will either start a new patient chart if the individual has never been there before, or pull that patient's chart out if he or she has previously used the store's services. Charts indicate prescriptions that have been filled before and types of frames purchased.

The optician will also take measurements of the distance between the centers of the pupils of the eyes to determine where and how lenses should be placed.

In choosing frames, the customer's occupation, hairstyle, and features must be considered. Other selection indications include the weight and thickness of the corrective lenses. The dispensing optician will help customers try on frames until they find one that looks good and feels comfortable. In some cases, especially with children or people who have never worn glasses, choosing frames can be a traumatic experience. The optician must put the customer at ease and be patient.

Once frames have been chosen, the optician will process a work order to give to the ophthalmic laboratory. This will include information on the lens prescription, size, and color as well as the frame type. In some cases dispensing opticians, trained in this area, may do the actual lab work.

When the glasses are ready, the optician checks the power of the lenses with various instruments to make sure that they are what has been prescribed and adjusts the frames to the customer's head so that the fit is perfect.

Opticians may also fit contact lenses for customers. Individuals must take specific measurements and prepare work orders much the same as they do with glasses. However, a great deal of skill and accuracy is needed when taking these measurements. Opticians must examine the contact lenses in the customer's eyes to make sure that they fit properly.

Dispensing opticians work various hours depending on the hours of the store or business and are responsible to either the owner, manager, or optometrist in charge.

Employment Opportunities

Dispensing opticians may be employed by:

- Optical chains or franchise stores
- Optical departments in department stores
- Optical departments in pharmacies
- Ophthalmologists
- Optometrists
- Privately owned optical shops

Expanding Opportunities for the Year 2000

As a result of the expanding middle-aged and older adult population who usually need some type of corrective lenses, there will be a growing demand for dispensing opticians.

The greatest number of job opportunities will be located in large metropolitan cities where there are more and larger optical shops and optical chain stores.

The biggest trend in this field is the one-stop shops for optical care where customers can have their eyes examined, choose frames, and have the glasses made within an hour.

Earnings

Earnings for dispensing opticians vary from approximately $15,000 to $35,000. Factors affecting salaries include the credentials, responsibilities, and experience of the individual. Other variables are the specific store, size, prestige, and geographic location where the dispensing optician works.

Individuals usually receive the highest salaries in states that require licensing. Dispensing opticians will also earn more working in larger, metropolitan cities.

Advancement Opportunities

Dispensing opticians can advance by obtaining additional training and experience. They may start out as apprentices and become full-fledged dispensing opticians. Others locate similar jobs in larger, more prestigious stores paying higher salaries.

Many dispensing opticians become managers of optical stores. Some become sales representatives for wholesalers or manufacturers of glasses, lenses, or frames. There are also individuals who go into business for themselves.

Education and Training

Education and training requirements for dispensing opticians vary from job to job and state to state. A great deal of the training is done on the job in the form of apprenticeship.

Formal training programs in opticianry are offered in community colleges, colleges, and universities. Only some of these programs are accredited by the Commission on Opticianry Accreditation. Schools that are accredited award two-year associate degrees in ophthalmic dispensing.

Some dispensing opticians receive basic training through programs designed for ophthalmic laboratory personnel. These are offered by many vocational-technical schools and trade schools throughout the country. Duration varies from just a few weeks to a year. After completion, individuals may become dispensing optician apprentices.

Many people in this field are trained totally on the job. In states where licensing is required, individuals must usually register with the state as apprentices and train for two to five years. On-the-job training may be informal or consist of structured programs that include technical training as well as office management, bookkeeping, and sales.

Individuals who go through accredited programs in states requiring licensing may be allowed to take licensing exams soon after graduation. This allows them to eliminate all or most of the two-to-five-year apprenticeship.

Experience and Qualifications

Experience requirements vary from employer to employer. Trainee positions generally do not require any experience while higher-level jobs do.

Qualifications also vary depending on the state. Some require dispensing opticians to be licensed. In order to obtain this license, individuals must usually go through an apprenticeship program and take an examination. To keep the license, dispensing opticians may have to take continuing education courses.

For Additional Information: Individuals interested in careers as dispensing opticians can contact the Opticians Association of America (OAA) and the Commission of Opticianry Accreditation (COA) for more information.

TIPS

• Large chain stores may offer structured apprentice training programs. These provide excellent opportunities for individuals to receive good training.

• Jobs may be advertised in the newspaper's classified section under headings such as ''Dispensing Optician,'' ''Eye Care,'' ''Optical Department,'' ''Fashion Eye Glass Shop,'' ''Eyewear,'' or the names of optical stores.

• Send your resume with a short cover letter to the owners or managers of optical shops, optical chains or franchise stores, and ophthalmologists or optometrists.

• Walk into optical shops and optical chain or franchise stores and ask if there are any openings.

PHARMACIST

Job Description: Dispense prescribed medication; advise on use and side effects of medicines; recommend over-the-counter medicines; maintain accurate records of prescribed customer medications.

Earnings: $30,000 to $51,000+

Recommended Education and Training: Degree from accredited college of pharmacy.

Skills and Personality Traits: Knowledge of drugs and interactions; personable; reliability; computer skills.

Experience and Qualifications: Practical experience or internship; state licensing.

Job Description and Responsibilities

Pharmacists usually work in pharmacies. They are responsible for dispensing medicines and drugs that have been prescribed by physicians, dentists, and other health practitioners.

When filling prescriptions for customers, pharmacists usually explain procedures for using the drug; possible side effects; and other medications, foods, or elements to avoid when taking the medication. For example, some medications cause side effects if taken with milk. Others may lose their effectiveness when alcohol is consumed. The pharmacist must be aware of everything to avoid when taking a medication as well as all the side effects.

Pharmacists keep a record of patient's prescriptions on a computer or in a card file. This allows the pharmacist to determine which medications are being taken to see if they can be combined. This is especially important when a number of different physicians are all prescribing medicines.

Pharmacists may assist customers in choosing over-the-counter medicines for a variety of ailments including the common cold, athlete's foot, tooth pain, headaches, and backaches. Many times pharmacists refer customers to a physician for further assistance. They may also answer many health-related questions themselves. It is important that the pharmacist be aware of all the health care supplies and medical equipment sold in the store and be able to advise customers on which product best suits their needs.

They must keep accurate records of all prescriptions filled and payments received. Pharmacists may be responsible for billing insurance companies and health maintenance organizations. This must be done on a timely basis in order to obtain reimbursement.

In some states there are mandatory inventories of all narcotics, needles, and syringes. Depending on the situation they are working in, pharmacists may be responsible for ordering drugs, medical supplies, and equipment.

Other functions of pharmacists working in stores may include managing the pharmacy and the store, supervising store personnel, displaying items, taking cash for purchases, and talking with sales reps. Individuals working in hospitals or health care facilities might also be responsible for evaluating the use of certain drugs in patient care, offering patient education programs, teaching students, and performing administrative duties.

Pharmacists' hours vary depending on the setting they are working in. Some work nights and weekends. Those who own stores will usually work longer hours than employees. Pharmacists may be responsible to either the manager or owner of a store or the head of the pharmacy department if they are working in a hospital. Those who own their stores are responsible to themselves. However, they must keep their customers happy or the customers will go elsewhere. Pharmacists must follow all rules and regulations of the state and federal government regarding the dispensing of pharmaceuticals.

Employment Opportunities

Pharmacists can work in a variety of settings including:

- Pharmacies (community and chain stores)
- Pharmacy departments in supermarkets
- Pharmacy departments in department stores
- Hospitals
- Health maintenance organizations (HMO's)
- Home health agencies
- Clinics
- Nursing homes
- Extended care facilities

There are also pharmacists who specialize in various fields. These include the radiopharmacists who prepare and dispense radioactive pharmaceuticals. Another field of specialization is called pharmacotherapy. Pharmacists in this area work with physicians to determine drug therapy.

Expanding Opportunities for the Year 2000

Pharmacists will be required in more settings because of research and technological advances that are resulting in new drugs to prevent and treat diseases.

It is estimated that on the average, older people use twice as many prescription medications as younger people. With the population of senior citizens increasing, there will be a larger demand for pharmacists to fill these prescriptions. The need for pharmacists will be especially great in states hosting a large aging population.

Earnings

Pharmacists earn from $30,000 to $51,000 or more with an average salary of $33,000 to $45,000. Pharmacists who own their own store or belong to a partnership will have higher earnings.

Earnings vary greatly depending on the individual's experience, duties, and responsibilities as well as the specific type of position. Size, prestige, and geographical location of the pharmacy are also factors.

Advancement Opportunities

Pharmacists can advance in a number of different ways. They may gain experience and obtain jobs in larger or more prestigious settings. Others land supervisory positions such as store manager or pharmacy supervisor. Advanced positions in hospitals and health care facilities include director and assistant director of pharmacy services.

Many pharmacists move ahead by becoming owners or part owners of pharmacies.

Education and Training

Pharmacists must graduate from a college of pharmacy accredited by the American Council on Pharmaceutical Education. The minimum requirement for pharmacists includes attendance of at least five years of college resulting in a Bachelor of Science or a Bachelor of Pharmacy degree.

Some individuals choose to obtain a Doctor of Pharmacy degree, or PharmD. A bachelor's degree is not required to enter this type of program. Instead, the aspiring pharmacist will go through six years of school in a combined bachelor's and doctoral program. (A bachelor's degree is not awarded.) Those who choose to obtain a bachelor's first may also go on for a doctoral degree, but it will usually take longer.

Individuals can also obtain a Master of Science degree in pharmacy if they are interested in research, teaching, or administrative positions.

Entrance requirements to colleges of pharmacy vary. Some schools require individuals to take the Pharmacy College Admissions Test (P-CAT). Others require up to two years of prepharmacy education in an accredited two-year school, college, or university. Some schools will admit students after graduation from high school.

Experience and Qualifications

All pharmacists must be licensed in the state in which they are working. Most states offer reciprocity. Individuals applying for a license must be at least 21 years old and demonstrate good character. Other requirements include graduating from an accredited college of pharmacy, passing a state board examination, and obtaining either a certain amount of practical experience or going through an internship under the supervision of a licensed pharmacist.

In order to renew the license, many states mandate continuing education.

For Additional Information: Individuals interested in becoming pharmacists can obtain additional information by contacting the American Association of Colleges of Pharmacy (AACP), the American Society of Hospital Pharmacists (ASHP), and the National Association of Boards of Pharmacy (NABP).

TIPS

• You might talk to pharmacists to learn more about their job and the field in general.

• Interview for several jobs before accepting one. Duties and responsibilities will be different in various settings.

• Large chain stores and major health care facilities often offer better benefits than small community pharmacies.

RADIOLOGIC TECHNOLOGIST

Job Description: Operate radiologic and imaging equipment; prepare patients for procedures; adjust equipment.

Earnings: $17,000 to $35,000

Recommended Education and Training: Formal training varies; most common training is a 24-month program leading to an associate degree.

Skills and Personality Traits: Compassion; communication skills; understanding of medical terminology; personable.

Experience and Qualifications: Licensing necessary in some states; certification and registration preferred.

Job Description and Responsibilities

Until a number of years ago, radiologic technologists used mostly X-ray equipment to determine broken bones and the extent of injuries, and to diagnose various illnesses. Today, modern technology has increased the various radiologic and imaging equipment and techniques used in health care to include ultrasound machines, magnetic resonance scanners, positron emission scanners, and more. As a result, the role of radiologic technologists is expanding.

The radiologic technologist is responsible for preparing patients for radiological tests. The individual will explain the technique to be used and answer any questions. The technologist is responsible for making sure that patients have removed all jewelry or other metal objects that would interfere with X-rays or other radiologic pictures.

For some procedures, the technologist will prepare a contrast medium for the patient to drink before having a procedure. When the patient drinks the medium, the radiologist can follow its flow through the body with images created on a screen. The radiologic technologist will assist the physician during this procedure by readjusting the patient's body and taking radiographs at the appropriate times.

The radiologic technologist is responsible for determining the correct distance and angle of the equipment in relation to the patient's body as well as the desired exposure time. Because too much radiation can be dangerous, it is important to use only as much as necessary to create a clear picture. Once images have been taken, the radiologic technologist is responsible for processing the film and getting it ready for the radiologist to read.

Other methods of imaging use ultrasound waves. Radiologic technologists who administer this type of procedure may be called sonographers or ultrasound technologists. The sonogram is widely used on pregnant women to determine the position, size, and health of the fetus. It is used for other procedures as well, such as diagnosis of tumors and cysts.

Another method of imaging uses magnetic fields instead of radiation or sound waves. This is called magnetic resonance imaging (MRI). This process is becoming increasingly popular for diagnosis of various illnesses.

The radiologic technologist must have a physician's order to perform any imaging techniques or procedures. The individual must keep records of all patients seen and procedures completed.

Radiologic technologists are usually responsible to the director of the radiology department if they are working in a health care facility or a physician if they are working in a doctor's office setting.

Employment Opportunities

Full- and part-time jobs are available for qualified radiologic technologists throughout the country. Individuals can work in a variety of health care situations including:

- Hospitals
- Mobile imaging clinics
- Physicians' offices
- Health maintenance organizations (HMO's)
- Diagnostic imaging centers
- Radiological groups
- Nursing homes
- Extended care treatment facilities

Expanding Opportunities for the Year 2000

As a result of the growing number of older people in this country, there will be a need for radiologic technologists who have specialized training working with the nonradioactive imaging techniques such as MRI's and ultrasound. Many diseases more prominent in aging people use these techniques for diagnostic purposes.

There will also be a need for radiologic technologists trained in radiation therapy.

Earnings

Annual earnings for full-time radiologic technologists range from approximately $17,000 to $35,000, depending on the specific health care facility as well as its size, prestige, and geographic location. Other factors include the responsibilities, experience, and training of the technologist. As a rule, the more specialized the training of the individual, the higher the salary.

Advancement Opportunities

Radiologic technologists can advance by obtaining additional or more specialized training. Individuals may then move into positions of specialization in the facility that they are currently working in or another larger or more prestigious facility.

Radiologic technologists may also advance their careers by assuming supervisory positions.

Education and Training

Education and training programs vary with the specialty. Prerequisites usually include a high school diploma or equivalency. The most common training program for radiologic technologists specializing in X-ray technology usually consists of a twenty-four-month course of study in radiography leading to an associate degree in applied science. There are, however, four-year programs that lead to bachelors' degrees or shorter programs that award certificates upon completion.

Radiologic technologists interested in specializing in sonography may take a one-year program in diagnostic medical sonography and receive a certificate.

Radiologic technologists who would like to specialize in the field of magnetic resonance imaging (MRI) may be trained by the equipment manufacturer of the MRI machine. Some hospitals also provide training programs for this specialty.

There are also one-year certificate programs that individuals already working in the health care field can use to obtain specialized training.

Experience and Qualifications

The necessity of the licensing is determined by the specific state in which individuals are working.

Professional credentials or registration in the field may be preferred for some jobs. Registration for radio-logical technologists is done by the American Registry of Radiologic Technologists (ARRT). Individuals specializing in sonography may be certified by the American Registry of Diagnostic Medical Sonographers (ARDMS).

For Additional Information: There are a number of organizations and associations that provide career information for radiologic technologists. These include the American Society of Radiologic Technologists (ASRT), the Society of Diagnostic Medical Sonographers, the Division of Allied Health Education and Accreditation of the American Medical Association, the American Registry of Radiologic Technologists (ARRT), and the American Registry of Diagnostic Medical Sonographers (ARDMS).

TIPS

• Not all hospitals have MRI equipment. If the facility you are working in does not have the machinery, you might want to contact a manufacturer to learn about training opportunities.

• Job openings are frequently advertised in the newspaper classified section under headings of "Radiology," "Radiologic Technologist," "X-Ray," "Sonographers," "Ultra-Sound," "Mobile Imaging Clinics," "Health Care," "Health Maintenance Organizations," "Diagnostic Imaging Centers," etc.

• After you have obtained general training, you can improve your career opportunities by continuing to take courses in specialized fields.

• Many cities have employment agencies specializing in the health care field.

PHYSICAL THERAPIST

. . . .

Job Description: Evaluate patients' physical therapy needs; perform physical therapies.

Earnings: $19,000 to $55,000 +

Recommended Education and Training: Bachelor's degree in physical therapy, master's degree, or certificate program.

Skills and Personality Traits: Mechanical aptitude; physical stamina; patience; communication skills.

Experience and Qualifications: Experience in physical therapy setting helpful.

Job Description and Responsibilities

Physical therapy is used for a number of purposes. These include helping people to ease pain and recover from injuries, accidents, or illness. Therapy can also help people regain the use of body parts. Patients may be born with physical disabilities or become disabled through strokes, heart attacks, accidents, or sports injuries.

Physical therapists evaluate and assess the therapy needs of patients and then develop, prescribe, and perform these procedures.

After evaluating a patient and performing a range of procedures, the physical therapist must reevaluate the therapy. If it is helping, the individual may continue the same routines; if not, the therapy may be revised. The therapeutic plan of care may take a few weeks, a few months, or many years, depending on the severity of the problem.

During the course of his or her work, the physical therapist will come in contact with a variety of rehabilitative personnel including physiatrists, physical therapy assistants, and physical therapy aides. In some situations, the therapist will give instructions to assistants and aides to carry out. In others, he or she will illustrate therapies directly to the patients or their families so that they can be done at home.

Physical therapists are responsible for keeping records and other documentation on patients. These records chart progress and therapies used.

Other duties of the physical therapist may include participating in conferences with the patient and his or her family, and the nursing staff and/or a social services department representative. If the therapist is in a supervisory position, he or she may also be required to order necessary equipment, schedule daily work loads, assess departmental needs, and assist in the maintenance of the physical environment of the therapy department.

As most facilities schedule appointments during the day, physical therapists usually work fairly normal hours. There are, however, some facilities that have therapists on staff 24 hours a day. Others may schedule sessions during the evening hours or on weekends.

Employment Opportunities

Qualified physical therapists will be able to find employment opportunities in almost every type of health care facility including:

- Hospitals
- Rehabilitation centers
- Nursing homes
- Extended care facilities
- Sports medicine clinics
- Private practice
- Independent physical therapy centers

Expanding Opportunities for the Year 2000

The current shortage of qualified physical therapists is expected to continue. Trends indicate that there will be an especially high demand in hospitals and extended care facilities.

Earnings

Earnings for physical therapists vary greatly depending on the specific facility, its size, prestige, and the geographical location in which an individual is working. Other variables include the responsibilities, experience, and education of the physical therapist.

Annual salaries range from $19,000 to $55,000 plus. Compensation is usually augmented by liberal benefit packages.

Advancement Opportunities

One way physical therapists can advance their careers is by becoming physical therapy supervisors. Another is to locate a similar position in a larger, more prestigious facility. This will result in increased earnings and responsibilities. Some physical therapists enter private practice as a method of climbing the career ladder.

Education and Training

A physical therapist is required to be a graduate of an approved school of physical therapy. Requirements vary for the type of degree the therapist must hold, depending on the position and state regulations. Individuals may need a bachelor of science degree or a master's degree with a major in physical therapy or a certificate from a licensed school. Many career changers who have bachelor's degrees in other subjects opt for the certificate program. Physical therapists must pass an examination after graduation to be registered and licensed.

Experience and Qualifications

Experience working in a physical therapy setting is useful. This experience may be obtained by working as a physical therapy assistant or aide. Hands-on experience in school is also useful.

Many states require that physical therapists be licensed. Check with individual states to determine specific licensing requirements.

For Additional Information: The American Physical Therapy Association (APTA) provides educational guidance and support for people in the physical therapy field.

TIPS

• Openings for physical therapists are advertised in the classified section of newspapers under headings such as "Physical Therapy," "Therapists," "Health Care," "Hospitals," and "Sports Medicine."

• Send your resume and a short cover letter requesting an interview to the personnel department of hospitals and other health care facilities. Ask that they keep your resume on file if a position is not currently available.

• Contact the placement office of the college you are attending (or have attended) to find out about job possibilities.

• There are a number of employment agencies around the country specializing in the health care industry.

PHYSICAL THERAPY ASSISTANT

Job Description: Assist physical therapist; administer therapy; handle paperwork.

Earnings: $11,000 to $23,000

Recommended Education and Training: Associate degree from an accredited college.

Skills and Personality Traits: Compassion; positive attitude; enthusiasm; ability to follow instructions.

Experience and Qualifications: Health care experience is useful, but not required.

Job Description and Responsibilities

Physical therapy eases pain and helps people recover from injuries, accidents, and illnesses. It also helps those with physical disabilities or those who become disabled by strokes, heart attacks, accidents, etc.

Physical therapists are responsible for evaluating and assessing the therapy needs of patients and then developing, prescribing, and performing these procedures or therapies. Physical therapy assistants are the paraprofessionals who work with the health care professionals, assisting them in fulfilling their functions. They work under the supervision of physicians, physical therapists, physiatrists, and rehabilitation specialists.

One of the functions of a physical therapy assistant is to help the physical therapist or physiatrist evaluate new patients. The PT assistant may be given orders to put a patient through a specific battery of tests to learn the extent of the injury or problem.

One of the jobs of the physical therapy assistant is to help a patient not only ease the pain, but also learn how to deal with it. This may be accomplished by providing various treatments including heat therapy or hydrotherapy such as whirlpool baths or wet packs. After working with patients, the physical therapy assistant may help the physical therapist reevaluate them.

The individual will be required to handle a great deal of the paperwork including patient records concerning problems, capabilities, treatments, and progress.

Physical therapy assistants work fairly normal hours. Therapy sessions are usually scheduled during the day; however, some facilities require evening or nighttime shifts. The individual is responsible directly to the head physical therapist, physiatrist, or rehabilitation specialist depending on the institution where he or she is working.

Employment Opportunities

Due to a nationwide shortage of qualified physical therapists and physical therapy assistants, employment opportunities can be located almost anywhere in the country on a full-time or part-time basis. Most health care institutions have more than one physical therapy assistant on staff. Opportunities for physical therapy assistants are available in a variety of health care facilities including:

- Hospitals
- Rehabilitation centers
- Nursing homes
- Sports medicine clinics
- Independent physical therapy centers
- Extended care facilities

> ### *Expanding Opportunities for the Year 2000*
>
> **Jobs in this field are abundant and projections indicate that the strong demand will continue in the future.**

Earnings

Physical therapy assistants earn approximately $11,000 to $23,000 annually. Most full-time employees also receive benefits.

Variables affecting salaries include the specific size and prestige of the facility, and the geographic location an individual is working in as well as how great the demand for people in this field is at the time. Other factors affecting earnings include the PT assistant's education, experience, and responsibilities.

Advancement Opportunities

Opportunities for advancement are excellent for physical therapy assistants who want to continue their education. Individuals taking an additional two-year training program at a school with an accredited program in physical therapy can become full-fledged physical therapists.

Education and Training

The minimum educational requirement for most physical therapy assistants is an associate degree from an accredited college offering a physical therapy or physical therapy assistant program.

Experience and Qualifications

PT assistants must have the physical stamina to lift and move equipment and people. It is also imperative that people in this field feel comfortable working in a health care facility and around people who are ill. Before getting involved in a career in physical therapy, some individuals get volunteer or part-time experience working in health care facilities.

For Additional Information: Additional information for people interested in a career as a physical therapy assistant is provided by the American Physical Therapy Association (APTA). This organization provides educational guidance and professional support for people in the physical therapy field.

TIPS

- The placement office of an accredited college offering a program in physical therapy may be aware of openings.

- Openings for physical therapy assistants are often advertised in the classified section in the newspaper or professional trade journals. Look under headings such as "Physical Therapy," "Physical Therapy Assistant," "Therapists," "Paraprofessional," "Health Care," "Hospitals," or "Sports Medicine."

- Send your resume with a short cover letter to the personnel director of health care facilities in the geographic areas you want to work in.

MUSIC THERAPIST

Job Description: Use music to treat physical, mental, and/or emotional disabilities.

Earnings: $14,000 to $40,000+

Recommended Education and Training: Minimum of a bachelor's degree in music therapy; many positions require a master's degree.

Skills and Personality Traits: Ability to play a musical instrument and sing; compassion; comfort working with handicapped and/or emotionally disturbed patients.

Experience and Qualifications: Internship in music therapy.

Job Description and Responsibilities

Music therapists use music and musical activities to treat physical, mental, and/or emotional disabilities. Music therapy is often used with other alternative expressive art therapies to make a breakthrough with a patient when other therapies have failed.

The music therapist works with other health professionals including physicians, nurses, teachers, physical therapists, dance therapists, psychologists, and psychiatrists. Depending on the specific job and patient, the music therapist may have varied duties. Those who work in hospitals, nursing homes or extended care facilities may be responsible for bringing a group of patients together to sing for the facility staff and other patients. The goal with this type of exercise is to encourage patients to come out of their shells and build self-confidence.

The music therapist may be responsible for planning musical activities for one patient at a time or for a group. He or she may teach patients new tunes or play tapes to help withdrawn patients reminisce, remember, and get involved. The therapist may work with handicapped patients, attempting to give them a renewed sense of accomplishment.

As with most therapy, music therapists must realize that progress may be slow. The slightest amount of progress can mean a great deal to a patient and his or her family.

Employment Opportunities

There are more opportunities for music therapists than there are qualified people to fill positions. Music therapists work in a variety of situations including:

- Hospitals
- Rehabilitation centers
- Prisons
- Nursing homes
- Extended care facilities
- Schools
- Independent expressive arts therapy centers

Expanding Opportunities for the Year 2000

As a result of the increasing aging population, there will be a great demand for music therapists in nursing homes, rehabilitation centers, and extended care facilities.

Earnings

Music therapists just entering the field can earn from $14,000 to $17,000 annually. Those who work at larger facilities and have experience may earn from $21,000 to $30,000. Supervisory positions in the field offer annual earnings of $40,000 and up.

Advancement Opportunities

Therapists can advance by obtaining supervisory or administrative positions. This type of advancement, however, limits the contact a therapist has with patients. Music therapists can also locate a position in research or teaching. Another option to consider is private practice or consulting.

Education and Training

Music therapists must have at least a bachelor's degree in music therapy. Some positions require a master's degree. Courses usually include music theory, voice studies, instrument lessons, psychology, sociology, and biology. Those who aspire to work in the public school system must also have a teaching degree.

Experience and Qualifications

Music therapists must be licensed in order to work in most positions. Licensing requirements include a six-month internship program. Individuals may gain additional experience by working at health care facilities or schools part-time or in voluntary positions.

For Additional Information: To learn more about the music therapy field, contact the National Association for Music Therapy, Inc. (NAMT) and the American Association for Music Therapy (AAMT).

TIPS

• Positions for music therapists are available through the federal government. Contact your state's employment service for more information.

• Register with the placement service offered by the National Association for Music Therapy, Inc. and the American Association for Music Therapy.

• Jobs may be advertised in the classified section of newspapers under "Music Therapist," "Health Care," "Expressive Arts Therapist," or "Therapy."

DANCE THERAPIST
• •

Job Description: Use dance to treat physical, mental, and/or emotional disabilities.

Earnings: $14,000 to $55,000+

Recommended Education and Training: Master's degree necessary.

Skills and Personality Traits: Dance skills; compassion; ability to work with handicapped and disabled people.

Experience and Qualifications: Internship required.

Job Description and Responsibilities

A dance therapist uses dance, movement, and related activities to treat disabled and handicapped patients. The individual must have extensive knowledge and understanding of body movement and what it can accomplish. Dance therapy is often used with other expressive arts therapies to make a breakthrough with a patient who cannot be reached in any other way.

The function of a dance therapist is to provide a

patient with a means of expression. Dance therapists work with doctors, nurses, teachers, physical therapists, musical therapists, psychologists, and psychiatrists to help restore an individual's health.

Working with one patient at a time or a group, the individual may teach a variety of dance forms. The therapist may also have the patient move freely to observe his or her movements and facial expressions. It is important to realize that what works for one patient will not always help another.

This job can be very fulfilling. Watching a patient with an unhealthy emotional or physical status improve through the personal efforts of the therapist is very rewarding.

Employment Opportunities

Employment prospects are excellent for dance therapists. There are more positions for qualified individuals than people to fill them. Work settings include:

- Hospitals
- Extended care facilities
- Schools
- Psychiatric hospitals
- Mental health centers
- Rehabilitation centers
- Nursing homes
- Correctional facilities
- Expressive arts therapy centers

Expanding Opportunities for the Year 2000

As a result of the increasing aging population, jobs will be especially plentiful in extended care facilities and nursing homes.

Earnings

Dance therapists can earn between $14,000 and $55,000 plus. Average yearly salaries in this line of

work run between $30,000 and $37,000 and are usually augmented by benefits. Factors affecting earnings include the specific facility an individual is working for and its size, prestige, and geographic location as well as the individual's experience, responsibilities, and educational level.

Advancement Opportunities

With drive and determination, dance therapists can advance their careers by moving into supervisory positions such as director of recreation therapy or expressive arts therapy.

Therapists may locate similar positions at more prestigious facilities or go into private practice.

Education and Training

A dance therapist must hold a master's degree in order to be employed in most facilities. Educational requirements for dance therapists are set by the American Dance Therapy Association (ADTA). This certifying group has approved the graduate programs of a number of colleges and universities throughout the country. If the individual does not attend one of the approved schools, the ADTA also has alternative education requirements.

Dance therapists hold undergraduate degrees in a variety of areas including liberal arts, dance, psychology, or physical education.

Experience and Qualifications

Dance therapists must be registered with the American Dance Therapy Association for most positions. In order to be registered, a dance therapist must fulfill certain educational requirements and obtain practical experience. This is usually achieved through an approved internship program.

For Additional Information: The American Dance Therapy Association (ADTA) provides educational and professional support and guidance to members as well as individuals interested in becoming dance therapists. It is also the registering agency for people in this profession.

TIPS

- Job openings are advertised in the classified section of the newspaper under headings of "Dance Therapy,"

"Health Care," "Therapists," "Recreation Therapy," "Expressive Arts Therapists," etc.

- The state and federal governments often have openings for dance therapists. These are usually civil service jobs and can be located through your state or federal employment service.

- Make sure you register with your college's job placement office.

VETERINARY TECHNICIAN

Job Description: Assist veterinarian in care of animals; collect specimens; assist in surgery; monitor improvement.

Earnings: $15,000 to $25,000

Recommended Education and Training: Associate degree in animal technology or applied science.

Skills and Personality Traits: Enjoy working with animals; strong stomach; ability to follow orders; scientific aptitude.

Experience and Qualifications: Experience working with animals helpful; certification or state licensing may be required.

Job Description and Responsibilities

Individuals in this position assist veterinarians as nurses do physicians. Specific duties and responsibilities vary depending on the job.

Veterinary technicians handle many of the same tasks as veterinarians with the exception of diagnosing problems, performing surgery, and prescribing medication. Technicians do, however, assist in these functions. Technicians help prepare animals for surgery and assist with the anesthesia and during the surgery itself. They check to see that the animals are coming out of anesthesia properly and that their progress is going according to schedule. Technicians also administer medication under the direction of the veterinarian.

Veterinary technicians are sometimes called animal health technicians. They work closely with the animals, watching them and reporting any problems to the veterinarian. Individuals must keep tabs on the physical symptoms and well-being of the animals as well as their psychological attitude. While performing this task, technicians may comfort them, play with them, and give them extra or special attention.

Technicians may also be responsible for changing dressings, cleaning animals, or holding them while the veterinarian performs procedures. Individuals may be required to draw blood, administer tests, and collect specimens to check for heartworm, fleas, and ticks.

In some instances, technicians assist in managing the facility. Individuals may be required to schedule appointments, obtain case histories, keep records, and handle billing and bookkeeping. Other responsibilities include talking to owners to determine symptoms, explaining pre- or postsurgical care and clarifying instructions for medication, diet, or care.

Veterinary technicians are responsible to the veterinarian in charge of the facility. Hours will vary depending on the facility's schedule.

Employment Opportunities

Veterinary technicians can work full- or part-time in a variety of animal care settings including:

- Animal hospitals
- Animal shelters
- Private veterinary clinics
- Zoos
- Humane societies
- Sanctuaries
- Horse farms
- Kennels

Expanding Opportunities for the Year 2000

With the increased concern for animal welfare, there will be a demand for veterinary technicians working in animal shelters and humane societies.

Earnings

Veterinary technicians earn between $15,000 and $25,000 annually. Factors affecting salaries include the experience and duties of the individual as well as the type, size, prestige, and geographic location of the facility.

Veterinary technicians with a great deal of responsibility and experience working in facilities in metropolitan areas will have earnings towards the upper end of the scale.

Advancement Opportunities

Veterinary technicians can advance by locating similar positions in larger or more prestigious facilities where they can receive increased earnings and responsibilities. Individuals may also go back to school, obtain a four-year degree in veterinary technology, and become paraveterinarians.

Education and Training

The recommended education for veterinary technicians is a two-year associate degree in applied sciences with a major in animal technology from an accredited school. There are also four-year programs for individuals who want to earn bachelors' degrees.

Courses in the sciences are a major part of this program. Course work in veterinary physiology, anatomy, animal care and management, radiography, anesthetic nursing and monitoring, animal pharmacology, parasitology, chemistry, biology, and communications will all be included.

Experience and Qualifications

Over thirty states require certification or licensing for veterinary technicians. In order to obtain this, individuals must usually complete an accredited program of study and pass a written exam.

For Additional Information: Individuals interested in becoming veterinary technicians can contact the American Veterinary Medical Association (AVMA) for information and literature.

TIPS

- Many zoos, animal shelters, humane societies, and sanctuaries have internships. These offer you an opportunity to get hands-on experience working with animals.

- Openings are often advertised in the classified section of the newspaper under "Veterinary Technician," "Animals," "Small Animals," "Zoos," "Animal Shelters," etc.

- Send your resume with a short cover letter requesting an interview to veterinarian clinics, hospitals, and animal shelters.

GERIATRIC SOCIAL WORKER

Job Description: Work with aging clients, assessing their situation and problems; counsel clients on economic, social, personal, and psychological matters; refer clients to proper agencies and people.

Earnings: $16,000 to $40,000+

Recommended Education and Training: Minimum of a bachelor's degree; some positions require a graduate degree.

Skills and Personality Traits: Compassion; counseling skills; communication skills; good judgment; dependability; objectivity.

Experience and Qualifications: State licensing or registration; certification is available.

Job Description and Responsibilities

Older people often have unique problems and circumstances to deal with. Geriatric social workers assist aging people and their families when they have difficulties. A big part of their job is to help seniors lead more productive lives.

Geriatric clients may be assigned to social workers for a number of reasons. Individuals may ask for help or be referred by another agency or person. Clients may be ill or have a spouse that is sick. In some cases, the clients don't have any relatives and cannot handle problems on their own. They may need medical or financial help, assistance with food and nutrition, help locating housing, etc. Many geriatric social workers deal with clients who are in nursing homes, extended care facilities or hospitals. They may also work with clients who are still in their homes and want to remain there.

Geriatric social workers talk to clients, evaluate problems, and assist in finding solutions. They advise the elderly and their families on available services including long-term care, housing, medical help, nutrition, and transportation.

The geriatric social worker may be required to contact a number of different agencies to handle the problems of one patient. For instance, he or she might utilize the local office of the aging, Meals on Wheels, home health aides, and an adult day care facility. After contacting the appropriate agencies and people, the geriatric social worker must coordinate all services. Individuals are expected to monitor the situation to make sure the client and his or her problems do not fall through the cracks of society.

A great deal of this job revolves around the rights of the elderly client. Geriatric social workers are often expected to investigate cases. For example, the individual may investigate abuse in a nursing home or cases of elderly people who appear not to be getting proper nutrition or who are neglected.

Other duties of geriatric social workers include visiting clients at home, preparing reports on each client, and evaluating programs for the elderly.

This is a job that may be emotionally draining. Geriatric social workers, however, are usually rewarded with the knowledge that they are helping people who very often cannot help themselves.

Employment Opportunities

Geriatric social workers can work exclusively in the geriatric area or may specialize in this field and handle other types of cases as well. They may work full- or part-time. Employment settings include:

- Government agencies
- Social service agencies
- Community organizations
- Religious organizations
- Hospitals
- Nursing homes
- Extended care facilities
- Home health agencies
- Hospices
- Consulting and private practice

Expanding Opportunities for the Year 2000

While the services of social workers are required by many older people, those most in need are individuals on low incomes and living alone.

Earnings

Geriatric social workers can earn between $16,000 and $40,000, depending on a number of factors. These include the education, experience, and responsibilities of the individual as well as the specific employment setting and geographic location.

As a rule, social workers with more education are paid higher salaries. Individuals with experience or those working in metropolitan cities with a high cost of living will also earn more.

Advancement Opportunities

After obtaining experience and/or additional education, geriatric social workers can advance in a number of ways. Some individuals are promoted to managerial, administrative, or supervisory positions. Others climb the career ladder by teaching in colleges or universities.

More options include going into research and opening consulting firms.

Education and Training

The minimum education required for most geriatric social workers is a bachelor's degree. The best major is one in social work with an emphasis or speciality in gerontology. Other choices for majors include sociology or psychology with courses in gerontology.

A master's degree in social work may be required for some positions including jobs in research, administration, supervision, or management. A PhD will usually be necessary for teaching and may be required for certain research positions.

Experience and Qualifications

Geriatric social workers graduate with a BSW and go through 400 hours of supervised field experience. This prepares them to work right after graduation. The MSW degree has a similar requirement including 900 hours of supervised field instruction or an internship.

Individuals who graduate with other types of degrees may be required to intern or obtain experience in other ways.

Social workers in any field may be required to obtain state licensing or registration. Voluntary certification is available through the National Association of Social Workers.

For Additional Information: Additional information is available from the Association for Gerontology in Higher Education (AGHE), the Council on Social Work Education (CSWE), and the National Association of Social Workers.

TIPS

- Internships are especially helpful in this field. Contact social service agencies, the office for the aging, or the department of mental health for details.

- Job openings are often advertised in the newspaper

classified section under headings such as "Social Worker," "BSW Needed," "MSW Needed," "Geriatric Social Worker," etc.

• Many jobs in this field are located in state, county, or municipal government agencies. Contact your local state employment office for information.

GERIATRIC ASSESSMENT COORDINATOR

• •

Job Description: Assess the needs of geriatric patients; set up care plan; coordinate health services; handle paperwork.

Earnings: $20,000 to $45,000+

Recommended Education and Training: Bachelor's degree in social work with an emphasis on geriatrics; some positions require a master's degree.

Skills and Personality Traits: Compassion; interpersonal skills; organization; ability to work with elderly.

Experience and Qualifications: Experience working with the elderly.

Job Description and Responsibilities

Geriatric assessment coordinators, serving as part of a multidisciplinary team, meet with geriatric patients to assess their physical, emotional, and mental condition. This is accomplished through examinations, medical tests, and interviews with both the patient and often the patient's family.

Once the patient has been assessed, the geriatric assessment coordinator will be required to determine the needs of the individual and set up a plan of care. This may include coordinating the services of physicians, nurses, nurse practitioners, physical therapists, recreational therapists, occupational therapists, and others. It may also include services such as a hot meal program, senior transportation plans, or adult day care.

It is essential, if possible, that the patient be included in the decision-making process regarding his or her plan of care. The coordinator will meet with the patient, and sometimes a patient's family, to discuss important decisions. These may include living arrangements and medical problems.

Depending on the specific employment setting and its structure, the geriatric assessment coordinator may be required to provide continuing contact with the patient, checking that the care plan is being followed. The individual may be responsible for reassessing patients as their situations change.

Hours for geriatric assessment coordinators will vary depending on shifts. Individuals are expected to work overtime in crisis situations.

Employment Opportunities

Geriatric assessment coordinators can be employed in a number of settings including:

• Hospitals
• Nursing homes
• Extended care facilities
• Health maintenance organizations (HMOs)
• Hospices
• Geriatric clinics

Expanding Opportunities for the Year 2000

Geriatric assessment coordinator is a relatively new career option that will grow as a result of the increasing number of elderly people in society today.

Earnings

Geriatric assessment coordinators have annual salaries ranging from $20,000 to $45,000 or more depending on their education, training, expertise, and responsibilities. Other factors affecting earnings include the size, prestige, and location of the specific facility.

Generally, the more education and experience an individual has the higher the salary. Individuals just starting out earn between $20,000 and $32,000. Geriatric assessment coordinators with a great deal of experience and responsibility, working in large or prestigious facilities, will earn the highest salaries.

Advancement Opportunities

Geriatric assessment coordinators can advance their careers in a number of ways. With additional experience and education, individuals can locate jobs with more responsibility in larger or more prestigious facilities. Individuals may also become the director of a geriatric program.

Many geriatric assessment coordinators climb the career ladder by expanding the program they are currently working in to include specialties such as adult day care, respite, or care for Alzheimer's or stroke patients.

Education and Training

As this is a relatively new career, education requirements vary. The minimum requirement for a geriatric assessment coordinator is a bachelor's degree in social work with courses in gerontology. The best degree to have for this job is either a master's or PhD in gerontology. A master's degree in social work with an emphasis on gerontology is also a good choice.

Experience and Qualifications

There is currently no credentialing process for geriatric assessment coordinators. Individuals must, however, have experience dealing with elderly people. This may be obtained through internships or volunteer experience.

For Additional Information: Individuals interested in a career as a geriatric assessment coordinator can obtain more information by contacting the National Association of Private Geriatric Care Managers (NAPGCM), the American Geriatrics Society (AGS), or the Association for Gerontology in Higher Education (AGHE).

TIPS

• Send your resume and a short cover letter to the personnel directors of hospitals, nursing homes, extended care facilities, and health maintenance organizations.

• Job openings are often advertised in newspaper classified sections under the headings of "Geriatric Assessment Coordinator," "Geriatrics," "Health Care," etc.

• Colleges and universities offering majors in gerontology usually have placement offices that are aware of openings.

NURSING HOME ACTIVITIES DIRECTOR

Job Description: Plan and lead activities; develop care plan; develop budget.

Earnings: $12,000 to $33,000+

Recommended Education and Training: Requirements vary from job to job.

Skills and Personality Traits: Organizational skills; creativity; supervisory skills; communication skills; good interpersonal skills.

Experience and Qualifications: Credentialing available; state approval may be required.

Job Description and Responsibilities

Nursing home activity directors are responsible for the daily recreational activities of the residents and patients in nursing homes and other similar facilities.

Activity directors are expected to plan activities in a variety of areas. These activities must be developed for people with various levels of skill and capabilities. When a resident enters a nursing home facility, the activities director is required to develop a personalized care plan. Each resident will be assessed by the activities director to determine an appropriate program of activities. In doing so, it is essential that the activities director finds out past and current interests and present abilities.

The activities director will work with the residents to plan activities in which they would like to participate. Together, they develop a list of activities that are appropriate for the residents. In cases where residents are incapable of planning their own activities, the director is responsible for handling the task.

The activities director meets with an interdisciplinary care team on a regular basis. This team includes nurses, physicians, dietitians, social workers, occupational therapists, physical therapists, recreational therapists, and pharmacists.

The director is required to prepare notes on each resident on a periodic basis, detailing progress. This may be done quarterly or more frequently. Notes might include items such as the manner in which residents are adjusting to the facility and whether they are participating in activities.

Activities may encompass solo projects as well as group events. These may include games, dances, parties, cooking lessons, shopping trips, craft classes, sing-alongs, dance classes, reading time, and exercise classes. Birthday, holidays, and other special events may be celebrated. The extent and complexity of activities will depend on the interest and abilities of residents as well as the budget of the facility.

This type of job can be very rewarding. Individuals can often see the difference in the quality of residents' lives as they become involved in various activities.

Employment Opportunities

Activity directors in nursing homes may work in small or large facilities. Individuals may be employed in:

- Private nursing homes
- Public nursing homes
- State-run facilities
- Hospitals
- Extended-care facilities
- Long-term care facilities

Expanding Opportunities for the Year 2000

Careers in all phases of geriatric care are increasing as a result of the large senior population. With more people living longer, there is a greater demand for nursing homes and extended care facilities. Activities directors are needed to staff these facilities.

Earnings

Earnings for nursing home activity directors range from approximately $12,000 to $33,000 or more. Factors affecting earnings include the education, experience, and responsibilities of the individual as well as the size, prestige, and location of the facility.

As a rule, individuals with higher education, working in larger facilities, will earn more.

Advancement Opportunities

Nursing home activity directors can advance by locating positions in larger, more prestigious facilities. This will usually result in increased earnings and responsibilities.

Education and Training

Educational requirements for nursing home activity directors can vary. The minimum is a high school diploma and two years' experience working full-time in a geriatric setting.

Some facilities prefer that their nursing home activity directors hold associate or bachelor's degrees. Possible majors include occupational therapy, geriatrics, recreation therapy, therapeutic recreation, rehabilitation therapy, or social work.

Organizations and trade associations may offer comprehensive training courses, workshops, and seminars.

Experience and Qualifications

Experience requirements vary for nursing home activity directors. In many instances, if the individual has a college degree in a related area, experience requirements are waived.

Individuals can obtain experience working as activity staffers or in other facets of geriatric care. Some activities directors work in recreation in other fields before becoming involved in geriatrics.

Individuals may become certified through the National Council for Therapeutic Recreation Certification.

For Additional Information: Individuals interested in learning more about careers as nursing home activity directors can contact the National Association of Activities Professionals (NAAP), the National Council for Therapeutic Recreation Certification (NCTRC), the American Health Care Association (AHCA), the American Therapeutic Recreation Association (ATRA), and the National Therapeutic Recreation Society (NTRS).

TIPS

• Send resumes and cover letters to hospitals, nursing homes, adult homes, and extended care facilities indicating your experience and interest in a job.

• Positions may be advertised in the newspaper classified section under headings such as "Nursing Homes," "Extended Care Facilities," "Adult Homes," "Long-Term Care Facilities," "Activity Director," "Director of Activities," "Geriatric Activity Director," or "Geriatric Recreation Director."

• Get experience by volunteering at local senior centers, nursing homes, extended care facilities, or hospitals.

RECREATIONAL THERAPIST

· ·

Job Description: Develop activities; observe reactions to activities; monitor patient progress.

Earnings: $18,000 to $35,000

Recommended Education and Training: Bachelor's degree in therapeutic recreation.

Skills and Personality Traits: Compassion; personable; organized; communication skills; creativity; ability to work with elderly and disabled patients.

Experience and Qualifications: Supervised internship; some states require licensing and/or certification.

Job Description and Responsibilities

Recreational therapists work with mentally, physically, and emotionally disabled patients. They attempt to rehabilitate patients through the use of various activities. In some situations, supervised recreational activities help patients forget about their physical, mental, and/or emotional problems and focus on the activities.

Many patients of recreational therapists are older people. Other patients may be mentally disturbed, mentally retarded, or recovering substance abusers. Patients are referred to recreational therapists to increase mental stimulation or physical strength and coordination. They may need to achieve a higher level of confidence or self-esteem. Some need to learn how to express their feelings or manage stress.

When choosing activities, recreational therapists must determine the patients' interests. Choice of activities also reflects the physical and emotional problems of the patients. Activities include craft projects or lessons, exercises, theatrical skits, games, and field trips.

One of the recent activities that many recreational therapists are finding useful, especially in nursing homes, is bringing puppies and kittens to the facility. Therapists have found that even patients with severe problems react well to animals.

Recreational therapists may work with other therapists including music, dance, art, and occupational therapists as well as physicians, psychiatrists, psychologists, and social workers. Together the team of professionals determines how best to treat the patient.

The recreational therapist is expected to talk with the patient, family, and the other professionals involved to find out the mental, physical, and emotional status of the individual. The therapist can then plan appropriate activities.

Recreational therapists oversee the patients as they participate in the various activities. Over a time span, the therapist must determine if the patient is improving. For example, does the patient interact well with others, gain more self-confidence, become more assertive, express feelings in a more positive manner, or deal with stress better?

If a treatment is not working, the therapist will be expected to develop other activities.

Employment Opportunities

While many recreational therapists work with the elderly, there are also opportunities in community-based programs for the disabled or in special education school programs.

Employment settings for recreational therapists include:

- Nursing homes
- Extended care facilities
- Hospitals
- Adult day care programs
- Community mental health centers
- Prisons
- Residential facilities for the mentally retarded
- Residential facilities for substance abusers

Expanding Opportunities for the Year 2000

As a result of the increasing aging population, there will be a need for recreational therapists in all types of nursing homes, long-term care facilities, adult care centers, and hospitals.

Earnings

Earnings for recreational therapists can range from approximately $18,000 to $35,000. Variables affecting earnings include the specific employment setting and its size, prestige, and location. Other factors include the experience, responsibilities, and education of the therapist.

Therapists with more experience and education will earn higher salaries. Individuals just entering the field can earn between $18,000 and $26,000. Those with experience who are working in more prestigious facilities or in geographic locations with higher costs of living can earn between $25,000 and $35,000.

Advancement Opportunities

With additional experience and education, recreational therapists can be promoted to administrative, supervisory, or management positions. Individuals might also advance their careers by locating similar positions in more prestigious facilities.

Education and Training

Education and training requirements vary from job to job. The recommended education is a bachelor's degree in therapeutic recreation, recreational therapy, or recreation with an emphasis on therapeutic recreation.

The course of study includes classroom and clinical work in abnormal psychology, physiology, medical and psychiatric terminology, program design, management and professional issues, helping skills, clinical practice skills, human anatomy, characteristics of illnesses and disabilities, concepts of mainstreaming and normalization, assessment and referral procedures, professional ethics, and the use of adaptive and medical equipment.

A graduate degree may be required for administrative, managerial, or supervisory positions or those in research or teaching.

Experience and Qualifications

Recreational therapists must go through a 360-hour internship program in which they obtain the necessary experience to work on their own.

In a number of states, recreational therapists must either be licensed or certified. In order to be licensed, individuals must usually graduate from a regionally accredited program in therapeutic recreation or recreation with an emphasis on therapeutic recreation. Other qualifications include going through a supervised internship and taking and passing a state licensing examination.

Certification is obtained through the National Council for Therapeutic Recreation Certification.

For Additional Information: Individuals interested in a career as a recreational therapist can obtain additional information by contacting the National Council for Therapeutic Recreation Certification (NCTRC), the American Health Care Association (AHCA), the American Therapeutic Recreation Association (ATRA), and the National Therapeutic Recreation Society (NTRS).

TIPS:

- Jobs are often available in Veterans Administration medical centers. Contact the Veterans Administration for more information.

- Job openings are advertised in the newspaper's classified section under "Recreational Therapist," "Therapist," "Gerontology," "Nursing Home," "Activities Director," "Health Care," "Long-Term Care Facilities."

- Colleges and universities offering programs in therapeutic recreation usually maintain placement offices that are notified of job openings.

- Get on-the-job experience volunteering in a nursing home, hospital, or long-term care facility.

BIOCHEMIST

Job Description: Conduct basic research; collect data; perform and analyze experiments.

Earnings: $20,000 to $75,000+

Recommended Education and Training: Minimum of a bachelor's degree in biochemistry or chemistry.

Skills and Personality Traits: Aptitude for sciences; good math skills; communication skills; manual dexterity; curiosity.

Experience and Qualifications: Experience requirements vary.

Job Description and Responsibilities

The work of biochemists is part biology and part chemistry. Biochemists study the chemical composition of living systems including animals, plants, insects, viruses, and microorganisms. They attempt to understand the complex chemical combinations and reactions involved in a variety of life forces such as metabolism, reproduction, growth, and heredity.

Changes are occurring in scientific objectives. Scientists have been chiefly interested in determining causes and effects, that is, what series of reactions occurred in order for certain things to happen. Now biochemists are beginning to look more at how to control the things that happen.

Biochemists have a variety of duties, depending on their specific job and the industry in which they work. Biochemists in health-related fields or pharmacology may search for ways to diagnose, treat, and cure illnesses or for new and better pharmaceuticals.

Biochemists in agricultural chemical companies may be responsible for researching the effect of new pesticides and herbicides on the growth of plant life. Those working in the food industry research nutrients, supplements, preservation, and other factors in the development of foods.

Biochemists use various equipment in the course of their jobs. Technology has increased the efficiency and speed of many tests as new equipment is more sophisticated than ever and can identify compounds more accurately.

Other responsibilities of biochemists include preparing reports on experiments and tests and supervising laboratory personnel. An interesting potential of biochemical genetic research is the possibility that more genetic diseases may be predicted and treated through an understanding of how genes operate and enzymes function. For example, future research may find a way to treat the cells in an individual with diabetes so that the cells have the ability to produce insulin.

Biochemists usually work fairly normal hours. They will be expected to work overtime when a project must be completed or a deadline is near.

Employment Opportunities

Biochemists may work in a variety of employment settings. These include:

- Government agencies
- Pharmaceutical companies
- Agricultural chemical companies
- Colleges and universities
- Food manufacturers
- Feed manufacturers
- Consumer product manufacturers

Expanding Opportunities for the Year 2000

Biochemists will be in demand in the pharmaceutical, biotechnology, and environmental protection fields. One of the largest growth areas for biochemists will be in research on the prevention and cure of AIDS.

Earnings

Earnings for biochemists vary depending on experience, education, responsibilities, and the specific industry in which they work. Salaries can range from $20,000 to $75,000 or more.

Generally, the more education and experience individuals have, the higher their salaries. Individuals working for federal government agencies will usually earn less than their counterparts in the private sector.

Advancement Opportunities

Biochemists can advance in a number of ways. They may obtain experience and additional education and lo-

cate positions in large or prestigious companies. Advancement potential includes promotions to project director or head biochemist.

Many biochemists decide to go into research. Others become professors at colleges and universities.

Education and Training

Biochemists are required to hold a minimum of a four-year bachelor's degree in biochemistry or chemistry. Positions in teaching will usually require a graduate degree.

The American Chemical Society approves college and university programs in the chemistry field. In addition to basic biochemistry and chemistry courses, individuals should take classes in cell biology, biochemical methods, genetics, and research.

Experience and Qualifications

Experience requirements vary for biochemists depending on the specific position. There are many entry level jobs for biochemists. These positions are often filled by recent college graduates and offer on-the-job training programs in lieu of experience.

For Additional Information: Individuals interested in learning more about a career as a biochemist can contact the American Chemical Society (ACS), the American Institute of Chemists (AIC), the American Association for Clinical Chemistry (AACC), and the American Society of Biological Chemists (ASBC).

TIPS

- The American Chemical Society has a career service offering career information and guidance.

- Colleges and universities with biochemistry programs usually have placement offices that list openings.

- Jobs are advertised in the classified section of newspapers and trade journals.

2

The AHPAT

About the AHPAT

● ● ● ● ● ● ● ● ● ● ● ● ● ●

The Allied Health Professions Admission Test (AHPAT) is an aptitude test that is used as a screening tool for admission to many allied health education programs of various sorts. The AHPAT is administered by the Psychological Corporation of San Antonio, Texas, on four scheduled testing weekends at 64 testing centers throughout the United States and in Puerto Rico. Special testing arrangements can be made for applicants living more than 150 miles from any of these testing centers and for candidates requiring a special date or accomodations for a disability.

The AHPAT is not a universal exam required for admission to all allied health programs. A number of one- and two-year programs ask that applicants take the AHAT. Some programs require SAT or ACT scores; some rely entirely on grade point average, recommendations, and personal statements; a few require applicants to submit scores from standardized exams for admission to graduate programs, such as the GRE or MCAT; some require specialized entrance exams such as the Nursing School Entrance Exam or the Pharmacy College Admission Test (PCAT); and still others have developed their own exams to be administered to their own candidates.

However, over 400 colleges, universities, and hospital schools in nearly every state as well as in the District of Columbia, Puerto Rico, and Canada do require that their applicants submit scores on the AHPAT for admission to some of their allied health training programs. These programs may include:

Art Therapy

Biomedical Engineering

Blood Banking Technology

Cardiopulmonary Technology

Cardiovascular Perfusion Technology

Certified Laboratory Assistant

Chiropractic

Circulation Technology

Cytotechnology

Dental Hygiene

Diagnostic Sonography

Dietetics and Nutrition

Environmental Health

Health Educators

Hospital and Health Services Administration

Medical Assistant

Medical Communication

Medical Illustration

Medical Records

Medical Technology

Mental and Community Health Services

Midwifery

Music Therapy

Nuclear Medicine Technology

Nurse Anesthetist

Nursing

Occupational Therapy

Orthopedic Assistant

Orthotics and Prosthetics

Physical Therapy

Physician Assistant

Podiatry

Radiation Therapy

Radiologic Technology

Recreation Therapy

Respiratory Therapy

Social Work

Speech Pathology and Audiology

Surgical Technology

Visual Sciences

If a school to which you are applying requires that you take the AHPAT to gain admission to the program that interests you, the school will give you registration information and will tell you the date by which you must have completed the exam. For more information you may write to:

Allied Health Professions Admission Test
The Psychological Corporation
555 Academic Court
San Antonio, TX 78204-3956
or call (512) 554-8198.

The AHPAT exam is a multiple-choice exam of about 270 questions administered in five separately timed sections. The subjects of the exam are: Verbal Ability; Quantitative Ability; Biology; Chemistry; and Reading Comprehension. The total time in the test room is about four hours.

All exam questions are in the form of a problem, question, or incomplete statement followed by four answer choices. Each question has only one correct answer; all questions are weighted equally. The scoring system is a simple one. Each correct answer earns one point. There is no penalty for a wrong answer and no penalty for a skipped space. Separate raw scores (that is, number correct) are reported for each of the five subject areas. In addition the Psychological Corporation reports percentile rankings for each of the five scores. There are no score conversions and no scaling.

Obviously, since wrong answers do no harm to your score and every right answer counts, you should do your best to answer every question. Use the full-length sample exam in this book to learn to pace yourself.

On the actual exam, answer the questions in order so as not to risk marking answers in the wrong space on the answer sheet. However, do not dwell too long on questions that you find especially difficult. Eliminate the answer choices that you are certain are wrong and guess from among those choices remaining. You are permitted to write in the question booklet, so feel free to cross out the choices you have eliminated and to scribble little notes to yourself. Whenever you guess, mark the question number in the test booklet with a big question mark. If time permits when you have finished the section, go back and rethink the questions you have marked as guesses. Ideally, you should pace yourself to read and consider the answers to each question. But if time is about to run out and a few questions remain, go directly to the answer sheet and mark all the remaining questions with the same answer. By the law of averages, you should get some right.

The sample AHPAT that follows is not an actual exam. It is, however, closely patterned on the real thing in terms of style, level of difficulty, and length. It will give you a good foretaste of the exam you must take. Try to set aside a single three-and-a-half hour block of time to take the full exam in one sitting with only one short break. If that is impossible, divide the exam into no more than two time periods. Do not look at any answers until you have completed the entire exam. Then check your answers against the correct answer key. Following the answer key is a full set of explanatory answers. We strongly urge that you read all the explanations, not only the explanations to the questions that you answered incorrectly. Even though none of these questions is likely to appear on your exam, there is a great deal to be learned from the reasoning and the process behind each answer here.

There is no passing score on the AHPAT. Each school that receives scores makes its own decisions as to what scores are acceptable for the specific program. In general, if you answer fewer than 75% of the questions correctly in any section, you should consider reviewing notes and textbooks and, perhaps, consulting a trusted teacher for advice as to how to improve your skill in that area so that you can achieve a better score on the actual exam.

Sample Allied Health Professions Admission Test
Answer Sheet

• •

VERBAL ABILITY

1. Ⓐ Ⓑ Ⓒ Ⓓ	16. Ⓐ Ⓑ Ⓒ Ⓓ	31. Ⓐ Ⓑ Ⓒ Ⓓ	46. Ⓐ Ⓑ Ⓒ Ⓓ	61. Ⓐ Ⓑ Ⓒ Ⓓ
2. Ⓐ Ⓑ Ⓒ Ⓓ	17. Ⓐ Ⓑ Ⓒ Ⓓ	32. Ⓐ Ⓑ Ⓒ Ⓓ	47. Ⓐ Ⓑ Ⓒ Ⓓ	62. Ⓐ Ⓑ Ⓒ Ⓓ
3. Ⓐ Ⓑ Ⓒ Ⓓ	18. Ⓐ Ⓑ Ⓒ Ⓓ	33. Ⓐ Ⓑ Ⓒ Ⓓ	48. Ⓐ Ⓑ Ⓒ Ⓓ	63. Ⓐ Ⓑ Ⓒ Ⓓ
4. Ⓐ Ⓑ Ⓒ Ⓓ	19. Ⓐ Ⓑ Ⓒ Ⓓ	34. Ⓐ Ⓑ Ⓒ Ⓓ	49. Ⓐ Ⓑ Ⓒ Ⓓ	64. Ⓐ Ⓑ Ⓒ Ⓓ
5. Ⓐ Ⓑ Ⓒ Ⓓ	20. Ⓐ Ⓑ Ⓒ Ⓓ	35. Ⓐ Ⓑ Ⓒ Ⓓ	50. Ⓐ Ⓑ Ⓒ Ⓓ	65. Ⓐ Ⓑ Ⓒ Ⓓ
6. Ⓐ Ⓑ Ⓒ Ⓓ	21. Ⓐ Ⓑ Ⓒ Ⓓ	36. Ⓐ Ⓑ Ⓒ Ⓓ	51. Ⓐ Ⓑ Ⓒ Ⓓ	66. Ⓐ Ⓑ Ⓒ Ⓓ
7. Ⓐ Ⓑ Ⓒ Ⓓ	22. Ⓐ Ⓑ Ⓒ Ⓓ	37. Ⓐ Ⓑ Ⓒ Ⓓ	52. Ⓐ Ⓑ Ⓒ Ⓓ	67. Ⓐ Ⓑ Ⓒ Ⓓ
8. Ⓐ Ⓑ Ⓒ Ⓓ	23. Ⓐ Ⓑ Ⓒ Ⓓ	38. Ⓐ Ⓑ Ⓒ Ⓓ	53. Ⓐ Ⓑ Ⓒ Ⓓ	68. Ⓐ Ⓑ Ⓒ Ⓓ
9. Ⓐ Ⓑ Ⓒ Ⓓ	24. Ⓐ Ⓑ Ⓒ Ⓓ	39. Ⓐ Ⓑ Ⓒ Ⓓ	54. Ⓐ Ⓑ Ⓒ Ⓓ	69. Ⓐ Ⓑ Ⓒ Ⓓ
10. Ⓐ Ⓑ Ⓒ Ⓓ	25. Ⓐ Ⓑ Ⓒ Ⓓ	40. Ⓐ Ⓑ Ⓒ Ⓓ	55. Ⓐ Ⓑ Ⓒ Ⓓ	70. Ⓐ Ⓑ Ⓒ Ⓓ
11. Ⓐ Ⓑ Ⓒ Ⓓ	26. Ⓐ Ⓑ Ⓒ Ⓓ	41. Ⓐ Ⓑ Ⓒ Ⓓ	56. Ⓐ Ⓑ Ⓒ Ⓓ	71. Ⓐ Ⓑ Ⓒ Ⓓ
12. Ⓐ Ⓑ Ⓒ Ⓓ	27. Ⓐ Ⓑ Ⓒ Ⓓ	42. Ⓐ Ⓑ Ⓒ Ⓓ	57. Ⓐ Ⓑ Ⓒ Ⓓ	72. Ⓐ Ⓑ Ⓒ Ⓓ
13. Ⓐ Ⓑ Ⓒ Ⓓ	28. Ⓐ Ⓑ Ⓒ Ⓓ	43. Ⓐ Ⓑ Ⓒ Ⓓ	58. Ⓐ Ⓑ Ⓒ Ⓓ	73. Ⓐ Ⓑ Ⓒ Ⓓ
14. Ⓐ Ⓑ Ⓒ Ⓓ	29. Ⓐ Ⓑ Ⓒ Ⓓ	44. Ⓐ Ⓑ Ⓒ Ⓓ	59. Ⓐ Ⓑ Ⓒ Ⓓ	74. Ⓐ Ⓑ Ⓒ Ⓓ
15. Ⓐ Ⓑ Ⓒ Ⓓ	30. Ⓐ Ⓑ Ⓒ Ⓓ	45. Ⓐ Ⓑ Ⓒ Ⓓ	60. Ⓐ Ⓑ Ⓒ Ⓓ	75. Ⓐ Ⓑ Ⓒ Ⓓ

QUANTITATIVE ABILITY

1. Ⓐ Ⓑ Ⓒ Ⓓ	11. Ⓐ Ⓑ Ⓒ Ⓓ	21. Ⓐ Ⓑ Ⓒ Ⓓ	31. Ⓐ Ⓑ Ⓒ Ⓓ	41. Ⓐ Ⓑ Ⓒ Ⓓ
2. Ⓐ Ⓑ Ⓒ Ⓓ	12. Ⓐ Ⓑ Ⓒ Ⓓ	22. Ⓐ Ⓑ Ⓒ Ⓓ	32. Ⓐ Ⓑ Ⓒ Ⓓ	42. Ⓐ Ⓑ Ⓒ Ⓓ
3. Ⓐ Ⓑ Ⓒ Ⓓ	13. Ⓐ Ⓑ Ⓒ Ⓓ	23. Ⓐ Ⓑ Ⓒ Ⓓ	33. Ⓐ Ⓑ Ⓒ Ⓓ	43. Ⓐ Ⓑ Ⓒ Ⓓ
4. Ⓐ Ⓑ Ⓒ Ⓓ	14. Ⓐ Ⓑ Ⓒ Ⓓ	24. Ⓐ Ⓑ Ⓒ Ⓓ	34. Ⓐ Ⓑ Ⓒ Ⓓ	44. Ⓐ Ⓑ Ⓒ Ⓓ
5. Ⓐ Ⓑ Ⓒ Ⓓ	15. Ⓐ Ⓑ Ⓒ Ⓓ	25. Ⓐ Ⓑ Ⓒ Ⓓ	35. Ⓐ Ⓑ Ⓒ Ⓓ	45. Ⓐ Ⓑ Ⓒ Ⓓ
6. Ⓐ Ⓑ Ⓒ Ⓓ	16. Ⓐ Ⓑ Ⓒ Ⓓ	26. Ⓐ Ⓑ Ⓒ Ⓓ	36. Ⓐ Ⓑ Ⓒ Ⓓ	46. Ⓐ Ⓑ Ⓒ Ⓓ
7. Ⓐ Ⓑ Ⓒ Ⓓ	17. Ⓐ Ⓑ Ⓒ Ⓓ	27. Ⓐ Ⓑ Ⓒ Ⓓ	37. Ⓐ Ⓑ Ⓒ Ⓓ	47. Ⓐ Ⓑ Ⓒ Ⓓ
8. Ⓐ Ⓑ Ⓒ Ⓓ	18. Ⓐ Ⓑ Ⓒ Ⓓ	28. Ⓐ Ⓑ Ⓒ Ⓓ	38. Ⓐ Ⓑ Ⓒ Ⓓ	48. Ⓐ Ⓑ Ⓒ Ⓓ
9. Ⓐ Ⓑ Ⓒ Ⓓ	19. Ⓐ Ⓑ Ⓒ Ⓓ	29. Ⓐ Ⓑ Ⓒ Ⓓ	39. Ⓐ Ⓑ Ⓒ Ⓓ	49. Ⓐ Ⓑ Ⓒ Ⓓ
10. Ⓐ Ⓑ Ⓒ Ⓓ	20. Ⓐ Ⓑ Ⓒ Ⓓ	30. Ⓐ Ⓑ Ⓒ Ⓓ	40. Ⓐ Ⓑ Ⓒ Ⓓ	50. Ⓐ Ⓑ Ⓒ Ⓓ

BIOLOGY

1. Ⓐ Ⓑ Ⓒ Ⓓ   11. Ⓐ Ⓑ Ⓒ Ⓓ   21. Ⓐ Ⓑ Ⓒ Ⓓ   31. Ⓐ Ⓑ Ⓒ Ⓓ   41. Ⓐ Ⓑ Ⓒ Ⓓ
2. Ⓐ Ⓑ Ⓒ Ⓓ   12. Ⓐ Ⓑ Ⓒ Ⓓ   22. Ⓐ Ⓑ Ⓒ Ⓓ   32. Ⓐ Ⓑ Ⓒ Ⓓ   42. Ⓐ Ⓑ Ⓒ Ⓓ
3. Ⓐ Ⓑ Ⓒ Ⓓ   13. Ⓐ Ⓑ Ⓒ Ⓓ   23. Ⓐ Ⓑ Ⓒ Ⓓ   33. Ⓐ Ⓑ Ⓒ Ⓓ   43. Ⓐ Ⓑ Ⓒ Ⓓ
4. Ⓐ Ⓑ Ⓒ Ⓓ   14. Ⓐ Ⓑ Ⓒ Ⓓ   24. Ⓐ Ⓑ Ⓒ Ⓓ   34. Ⓐ Ⓑ Ⓒ Ⓓ   44. Ⓐ Ⓑ Ⓒ Ⓓ
5. Ⓐ Ⓑ Ⓒ Ⓓ   15. Ⓐ Ⓑ Ⓒ Ⓓ   25. Ⓐ Ⓑ Ⓒ Ⓓ   35. Ⓐ Ⓑ Ⓒ Ⓓ   45. Ⓐ Ⓑ Ⓒ Ⓓ
6. Ⓐ Ⓑ Ⓒ Ⓓ   16. Ⓐ Ⓑ Ⓒ Ⓓ   26. Ⓐ Ⓑ Ⓒ Ⓓ   36. Ⓐ Ⓑ Ⓒ Ⓓ   46. Ⓐ Ⓑ Ⓒ Ⓓ
7. Ⓐ Ⓑ Ⓒ Ⓓ   17. Ⓐ Ⓑ Ⓒ Ⓓ   27. Ⓐ Ⓑ Ⓒ Ⓓ   37. Ⓐ Ⓑ Ⓒ Ⓓ   47. Ⓐ Ⓑ Ⓒ Ⓓ
8. Ⓐ Ⓑ Ⓒ Ⓓ   18. Ⓐ Ⓑ Ⓒ Ⓓ   28. Ⓐ Ⓑ Ⓒ Ⓓ   38. Ⓐ Ⓑ Ⓒ Ⓓ   48. Ⓐ Ⓑ Ⓒ Ⓓ
9. Ⓐ Ⓑ Ⓒ Ⓓ   19. Ⓐ Ⓑ Ⓒ Ⓓ   29. Ⓐ Ⓑ Ⓒ Ⓓ   39. Ⓐ Ⓑ Ⓒ Ⓓ   49. Ⓐ Ⓑ Ⓒ Ⓓ
10. Ⓐ Ⓑ Ⓒ Ⓓ   20. Ⓐ Ⓑ Ⓒ Ⓓ   30. Ⓐ Ⓑ Ⓒ Ⓓ   40. Ⓐ Ⓑ Ⓒ Ⓓ   50. Ⓐ Ⓑ Ⓒ Ⓓ

CHEMISTRY

1. Ⓐ Ⓑ Ⓒ Ⓓ   11. Ⓐ Ⓑ Ⓒ Ⓓ   21. Ⓐ Ⓑ Ⓒ Ⓓ   31. Ⓐ Ⓑ Ⓒ Ⓓ   41. Ⓐ Ⓑ Ⓒ Ⓓ
2. Ⓐ Ⓑ Ⓒ Ⓓ   12. Ⓐ Ⓑ Ⓒ Ⓓ   22. Ⓐ Ⓑ Ⓒ Ⓓ   32. Ⓐ Ⓑ Ⓒ Ⓓ   42. Ⓐ Ⓑ Ⓒ Ⓓ
3. Ⓐ Ⓑ Ⓒ Ⓓ   13. Ⓐ Ⓑ Ⓒ Ⓓ   23. Ⓐ Ⓑ Ⓒ Ⓓ   33. Ⓐ Ⓑ Ⓒ Ⓓ   43. Ⓐ Ⓑ Ⓒ Ⓓ
4. Ⓐ Ⓑ Ⓒ Ⓓ   14. Ⓐ Ⓑ Ⓒ Ⓓ   24. Ⓐ Ⓑ Ⓒ Ⓓ   34. Ⓐ Ⓑ Ⓒ Ⓓ   44. Ⓐ Ⓑ Ⓒ Ⓓ
5. Ⓐ Ⓑ Ⓒ Ⓓ   15. Ⓐ Ⓑ Ⓒ Ⓓ   25. Ⓐ Ⓑ Ⓒ Ⓓ   35. Ⓐ Ⓑ Ⓒ Ⓓ   45. Ⓐ Ⓑ Ⓒ Ⓓ
6. Ⓐ Ⓑ Ⓒ Ⓓ   16. Ⓐ Ⓑ Ⓒ Ⓓ   26. Ⓐ Ⓑ Ⓒ Ⓓ   36. Ⓐ Ⓑ Ⓒ Ⓓ   46. Ⓐ Ⓑ Ⓒ Ⓓ
7. Ⓐ Ⓑ Ⓒ Ⓓ   17. Ⓐ Ⓑ Ⓒ Ⓓ   27. Ⓐ Ⓑ Ⓒ Ⓓ   37. Ⓐ Ⓑ Ⓒ Ⓓ   47. Ⓐ Ⓑ Ⓒ Ⓓ
8. Ⓐ Ⓑ Ⓒ Ⓓ   18. Ⓐ Ⓑ Ⓒ Ⓓ   28. Ⓐ Ⓑ Ⓒ Ⓓ   38. Ⓐ Ⓑ Ⓒ Ⓓ   48. Ⓐ Ⓑ Ⓒ Ⓓ
9. Ⓐ Ⓑ Ⓒ Ⓓ   19. Ⓐ Ⓑ Ⓒ Ⓓ   29. Ⓐ Ⓑ Ⓒ Ⓓ   39. Ⓐ Ⓑ Ⓒ Ⓓ   49. Ⓐ Ⓑ Ⓒ Ⓓ
10. Ⓐ Ⓑ Ⓒ Ⓓ   20. Ⓐ Ⓑ Ⓒ Ⓓ   30. Ⓐ Ⓑ Ⓒ Ⓓ   40. Ⓐ Ⓑ Ⓒ Ⓓ   50. Ⓐ Ⓑ Ⓒ Ⓓ

READING COMPREHENSION

1. Ⓐ Ⓑ Ⓒ Ⓓ   10. Ⓐ Ⓑ Ⓒ Ⓓ   19. Ⓐ Ⓑ Ⓒ Ⓓ   28. Ⓐ Ⓑ Ⓒ Ⓓ   37. Ⓐ Ⓑ Ⓒ Ⓓ
2. Ⓐ Ⓑ Ⓒ Ⓓ   11. Ⓐ Ⓑ Ⓒ Ⓓ   20. Ⓐ Ⓑ Ⓒ Ⓓ   29. Ⓐ Ⓑ Ⓒ Ⓓ   38. Ⓐ Ⓑ Ⓒ Ⓓ
3. Ⓐ Ⓑ Ⓒ Ⓓ   12. Ⓐ Ⓑ Ⓒ Ⓓ   21. Ⓐ Ⓑ Ⓒ Ⓓ   30. Ⓐ Ⓑ Ⓒ Ⓓ   39. Ⓐ Ⓑ Ⓒ Ⓓ
4. Ⓐ Ⓑ Ⓒ Ⓓ   13. Ⓐ Ⓑ Ⓒ Ⓓ   22. Ⓐ Ⓑ Ⓒ Ⓓ   31. Ⓐ Ⓑ Ⓒ Ⓓ   40. Ⓐ Ⓑ Ⓒ Ⓓ
5. Ⓐ Ⓑ Ⓒ Ⓓ   14. Ⓐ Ⓑ Ⓒ Ⓓ   23. Ⓐ Ⓑ Ⓒ Ⓓ   32. Ⓐ Ⓑ Ⓒ Ⓓ   41. Ⓐ Ⓑ Ⓒ Ⓓ
6. Ⓐ Ⓑ Ⓒ Ⓓ   15. Ⓐ Ⓑ Ⓒ Ⓓ   24. Ⓐ Ⓑ Ⓒ Ⓓ   33. Ⓐ Ⓑ Ⓒ Ⓓ   42. Ⓐ Ⓑ Ⓒ Ⓓ
7. Ⓐ Ⓑ Ⓒ Ⓓ   16. Ⓐ Ⓑ Ⓒ Ⓓ   25. Ⓐ Ⓑ Ⓒ Ⓓ   34. Ⓐ Ⓑ Ⓒ Ⓓ   43. Ⓐ Ⓑ Ⓒ Ⓓ
8. Ⓐ Ⓑ Ⓒ Ⓓ   17. Ⓐ Ⓑ Ⓒ Ⓓ   26. Ⓐ Ⓑ Ⓒ Ⓓ   35. Ⓐ Ⓑ Ⓒ Ⓓ   44. Ⓐ Ⓑ Ⓒ Ⓓ
9. Ⓐ Ⓑ Ⓒ Ⓓ   18. Ⓐ Ⓑ Ⓒ Ⓓ   27. Ⓐ Ⓑ Ⓒ Ⓓ   36. Ⓐ Ⓑ Ⓒ Ⓓ   45. Ⓐ Ⓑ Ⓒ Ⓓ

Sample Allied Health Professions Admission Test

VERBAL ABILITY

75 questions

Directions: For questions 1 to 35, choose the word that means the same or most nearly the same as the CAPITALIZED word.

1. DELINQUENT
   (A) youthful
   (B) lawless
   (C) late
   (D) violent

2. PROSCRIBE
   (A) explain
   (B) deny
   (C) publish
   (D) forbid

3. CLEMENCY
   (A) amnesty
   (B) rectitude
   (C) mercy
   (D) pardon

4. REHABILITATE
   (A) compensate
   (B) train
   (C) replace
   (D) restore

5. CURSORY
   (A) handwritten
   (B) flowing
   (C) superficial
   (D) profane

6. TACITLY
   (A) silently
   (B) concisely
   (C) delicately
   (D) tangibly

7. INDIGENT
   (A) deserving
   (B) angry
   (C) lazy
   (D) poor

8. STRINGENT
   (A) severe
   (B) harsh
   (C) unfair
   (D) cleansing

9. PECUNIARY
   (A) strange
   (B) financial
   (C) special
   (D) intense

10. TABULATE
    (A) systematize
    (B) count
    (C) total
    (D) file

11. FACSIMILE
    (A) forgery
    (B) scrap
    (C) copy
    (D) approximation

12. PERUSE
    (A) study
    (B) seize
    (C) stroll
    (D) spindle

13. LARCENY
    (A) burglary
    (B) robbery
    (C) embezzlement
    (D) theft

14. NOXIOUS
    (A) unpleasant
    (B) odoriferous
    (C) harmful
    (D) hysterical

15. APPRISE
    (A) notify
    (B) repeat
    (C) judge
    (D) warn

16. FISCAL
    (A) insufficient
    (B) final
    (C) inherited
    (D) financial

17. INTERIM
    (A) permanent
    (B) valueless
    (C) worthwhile
    (D) temporary

18. COLLABORATE
    (A) work rapidly
    (B) work together
    (C) work independently
    (D) work overtime

19. ALTRUISTIC
    (A) unselfish
    (B) extended
    (C) organized
    (D) appealing

20. FRAUDULENT
    (A) suspicious
    (B) deceptive
    (C) unfair
    (D) despicable

21. ALLEGATION
    (A) denial
    (B) response
    (C) inquiry
    (D) assertion

22. STIPULATION
    (A) essential specification
    (B) unnecessary addition
    (C) required training
    (D) required correction

23. ALLOCATION
    (A) prevention
    (B) site
    (C) exchange
    (D) assignment

24. PERENNIAL
    (A) changeable
    (B) frequent
    (C) occasional
    (D) enduring

25. EMISSIONS
    (A) discharges
    (B) embassies
    (C) approaches
    (D) trends

26. RHETORICAL
    (A) inquisitive
    (B) laconic
    (C) tacit
    (D) grandiloquent

27. RUDIMENTARY
    (A) classic
    (B) basic
    (C) remunerative
    (D) vertebrate

28. SALUTARY
    (A) popular
    (B) welcoming
    (C) beneficial
    (D) forceful

29. ACQUIESCE
    (A) endeavor
    (B) discharge
    (C) agree
    (D) inquire

30. DIFFIDENCE
    (A) shyness
    (B) distinction
    (C) unconcern
    (D) discordance

31. CAPITULATE
    (A) repeat
    (B) surrender
    (C) finance
    (D) retreat

32. AUSPICIOUS
    (A) questionable
    (B) well known
    (C) free
    (D) favorable

33. ACCESS
    (A) too much
    (B) extra
    (C) admittance
    (D) arrival

34. COGENT
    (A) confused
    (B) opposite
    (C) unintentional
    (D) convincing

35. OSTENSIBLY
    (A) undoubtedly
    (B) infrequently
    (C) powerfully
    (D) apparently

Directions: For questions 36 to 75, choose the word which means the opposite or most nearly the opposite of the CAPITALIZED word.

36. QUERY
    (A) argument
    (B) answer
    (C) square
    (D) loner

37. VITRIOLIC
    (A) benevolent
    (B) vanquished
    (C) invisible
    (D) alcoholic

38. MYOPIC
    (A) poisonous
    (B) toadstool
    (C) froglike
    (D) open-minded

39. NAPPED
    (A) awake
    (B) tired
    (C) soft
    (D) smooth

40. PLACATE
    (A) amuse
    (B) antagonize
    (C) embroil
    (D) pity

41. RETICENT
    (A) fidgety
    (B) repetitious
    (C) talkative
    (D) restful

42. ECLECTIC
    (A) brilliant
    (B) exclusive
    (C) prosaic
    (D) conclusive

43. EXPUNGE
    (A) clarify
    (B) embroil
    (C) perpetuate
    (D) investigate

44. AMBULATORY
    (A) supine
    (B) influential
    (C) injured
    (D) quarantined

45. PROCRASTINATE
    (A) eulogize
    (B) invest
    (C) expedite
    (D) insinuate

46. INTREPID
    (A) surreptitious
    (B) monotonous
    (C) theocratic
    (D) paranoid

47. CAUSE
    (A) affect
    (B) result
    (C) question
    (D) matter

48. PITHY
    (A) wooden
    (B) boring
    (C) inane
    (D) bareheaded

49. RURAL
    (A) suburban
    (B) exurban
    (C) arid
    (D) urban

50. BIRTH
    (A) life
    (B) age
    (C) childlessness
    (D) death

51. HUMANE
    (A) bestial
    (B) ill-mannered
    (C) ill-tempered
    (D) anthropomorphic

52. HARD
    (A) crisp
    (B) soft
    (C) wet
    (D) weak

53. ACID
    (A) sweet
    (B) bitter
    (C) bland
    (D) alkaline

54. BRUSQUE
    (A) patient
    (B) clean
    (C) dirty
    (D) dusty

55. ABSTRACT
    (A) art
    (B) absurd
    (C) sculpture
    (D) concrete

56. ANOREXIA
    (A) brazenness
    (B) gluttony
    (C) disrespect
    (D) anarchy

57. CEILING
    (A) roof
    (B) wall
    (C) floor
    (D) foundation

58. FISSION
    (A) fusion
    (B) rendition
    (C) confiscation
    (D) absolution

59. FREEZE
    (A) hot
    (B) bend
    (C) slow
    (D) water

60. PROVINCIAL
    (A) urbane
    (B) rootless
    (C) untroubled
    (D) temporary

61. SECULAR
    (A) whole
    (B) combined
    (C) clerical
    (D) educational

62. VERVE
    (A) cowardice
    (B) ability
    (C) lethargy
    (D) litany

63. GLUTINOUS
   (A) slick
   (B) swollen
   (C) hungry
   (D) lurid

64. GROTTO
   (A) giant
   (B) child
   (C) desert
   (D) mound

65. VERDANT
   (A) barren
   (B) untruthful
   (C) reckless
   (D) obnoxious

66. TREPIDATION
   (A) fearlessness
   (B) anger
   (C) honesty
   (D) vigor

67. RESCIND
   (A) provide
   (B) reinstate
   (C) cancel
   (D) mutilate

68. ABATEMENT
   (A) addition
   (B) guarantee
   (C) denial
   (D) danger

69. OFFICIOUS
   (A) informal
   (B) illegal
   (C) aloof
   (D) bureaucratic

70. DOVE
   (A) eagle
   (B) hawk
   (C) turkey
   (D) ostrich

71. ADULTERATED
   (A) immature
   (B) disgraced
   (C) pure
   (D) destroyed

72. STAMINA
   (A) fatigue
   (B) nerve
   (C) pistil
   (D) disgrace

73. SUPPLE
   (A) soft
   (B) stale
   (C) lazy
   (D) rigid

74. CATHARSIS
   (A) rowboat
   (B) argument
   (C) success
   (D) repression

75. NEPOTISM
   (A) impartiality
   (B) demagogy
   (C) indifference
   (D) apathy

End of Verbal Ability Section

If you finish your work on this section before time is called, check over your work on this section only. Do not continue to the next section until the signal is given.

QUANTITATIVE ABILITY

50 questions

Directions: Solve each problem and choose the best answer.

1. Which of the following is the quotient of 333,180 and 617?

   (A) 541

   (B) 542

   (C) 549

   (D) 540

2. The fraction $^{432}/_{801}$ can be reduced by dividing numerator and denominator by

   (A) 2

   (B) 4

   (C) 6

   (D) 9

3. The value of $3° + 9^{1/2} + (1/3)^{-2}$ is

   (A) $1\frac{1}{2}$

   (B) $3\frac{1}{2}$

   (C) 5

   (D) 13

4. The temperatures reported at hour intervals on a winter evening were $+4°$, $0°$, $-1°$, $-5°$, and $-8°$. Find the average temperature for these hours.

   (A) $-10°$

   (B) $-2°$

   (C) $+2°$

   (D) $-2\frac{1}{2}°$

5. If the radius of a circle is increased by 3, the circumference is increased by

   (A) 3

   (B) 3π

   (C) 6

   (D) 6π

6.

TRIGONOMETRIC VALUES

Angle	Sin	Cos	Tan
58°	.8480	.5299	1.6003
59°	.8572	.5150	1.6643
60°	.8660	.5000	1.7321
61°	.8746	.4848	1.8040
62°	.8829	.4695	1.8807
63°	.8910	.4540	1.9626
64°	.8988	.4384	2.0503
65°	.9063	.4226	2.1445
66°	.9135	.4067	2.2460
67°	.9205	.3907	2.3559
68°	.9272	.3746	2.4751
69°	.9336	.3584	2.6051
70°	.9397	.3420	2.7475
71°	.9455	.3256	2.9042
72°	.9511	.3090	3.0777
73°	.9563	.2924	3.2709

If $\cos \angle A = .4000$, find $\angle A$ to the nearest degree.

   (A) 66°

   (B) 67°

   (C) 68°

   (D) 69°

7. Subtract $^3/_5$ from $^9/_{11}$.

   (A) $-^{12}/_{55}$

   (B) $^{12}/_{55}$

   (C) 1

   (D) $^3/_8$

8. Subtract $\dfrac{6x + 5y}{2x} - \dfrac{4x + y}{2x}$

   (A) $1 + 4y$

   (B) $4y$

   (C) $1 + 2y$

   (D) $\dfrac{x + 2y}{x}$

9. Combine $4\sqrt{27} - 2\sqrt{48} + \sqrt{147}$

   (A) $27\sqrt{3}$

   (B) $-3\sqrt{3}$

   (C) $9\sqrt{3}$

   (D) $11\sqrt{3}$

10. In a parallelogram whose area is 15, the base is represented by $x + 7$ and the altitude is $x - 7$. Find the base of the parallelogram.

    (A) 8

    (B) 15

    (C) 1

    (D) 34

11. Use the Trigonometric Values in the table accompanying question 6 to answer question 11.

    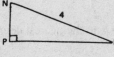

    If $\angle N = 68°$ and $MN = 4$, then to the nearest tenth, $NP =$

    (A) .1

    (B) .8

    (C) 1.5

    (D) 6.8

12. Find $\tfrac{7}{8} \cdot \tfrac{2}{3} \div \tfrac{1}{8}$.

    (A) $\tfrac{3}{14}$

    (B) $\tfrac{7}{96}$

    (C) $\tfrac{21}{128}$

    (D) $\tfrac{14}{3}$

13. Find the product of $(2x - 3)$ and $(3x + 5)$.

    (A) $6x^2 + 15$

    (B) $16x^2 - 24x$

    (C) $6x^2 - 15$

    (D) $6x^2 + x - 15$

14. Subtract $45\tfrac{5}{12}$ from 61.

    (A) $15\tfrac{7}{12}$

    (B) $15\tfrac{5}{12}$

    (C) $16\tfrac{7}{12}$

    (D) $16\tfrac{5}{12}$

15. Multiply and simplify: $2\sqrt{18} \cdot 6\sqrt{2}$

    (A) 72

    (B) 48

    (C) $12\sqrt{6}$

    (D) $8\sqrt{6}$

16. A class had these grades on a quiz:
    9, 10, 7, 9, 5, 7, 8, 0, 4, 7, 1, 5, 5, 4, 10, 4, 7
    The median of the grades is

    (A) 5

    (B) 6

    (C) 6.5

    (D) 7

17. Using the information in question 16 above, the mode of the grades is

    (A) 5

    (B) 6

    (C) 6.5

    (D) 7

18. A cylindrical pail has a radius of 7 inches and a height of 10 inches. Approximately how many gallons will the pail hold, if there are 231 cubic inches to a gallon? (Use $\pi = \tfrac{22}{7}$.)

    (A) .9

    (B) 4.2

    (C) 6.7

    (D) 5.1

19. In triangle ABC, ∡C is a right angle. If sin A = ½, what is the value of sin B?

(A) $\dfrac{\sqrt{3}}{2}$

(B) $\sqrt{3}$

(C) $\dfrac{\sqrt{3}}{3}$

(D) ½

20. Which of the following fractions is closest to ½?

(A) $5/12$

(B) $8/15$

(C) $7/15$

(D) $31/60$

21. If AB is parallel to CD and angle 1 = x°, then the sum of angle 1 and angle 2 is

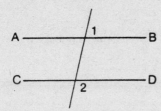

(A) 2x°

(B) (180 − x)°

(C) 180°

(D) (180 + x)°

22. 2(a - b) + 4(a + 3b) =

(A) 6a + 10b

(B) 6a + 2b

(C) 6a − 10b

(D) $8a^2 + 2b^2$

23. Reduce to lowest terms: $\dfrac{3x^3 - 3x^2y}{9x^2 - 9xy}$

(A) $\dfrac{x}{6}$

(B) $\dfrac{x}{3}$

(C) $\dfrac{2x}{3}$

(D) 1

24. Write $5/12$ as an equivalent percent.

(A) 41%

(B) 41.6%

(C) 41⅔%

(D) 4.1%

25. The angles of a triangle are in the ratio 1:5:6. This triangle is

(A) acute

(B) obtuse

(C) isosceles

(D) right

26. What part of an hour elapses between 3:45 P.M. and 4:09 P.M.?

(A) $6/25$

(B) $2/5$

(C) $5/12$

(D) $1/24$

27. Find the average of the first 5 positive integers that end in 3.

(A) 3

(B) 13

(C) 18

(D) 23

28. The number of degrees in angle ABC is

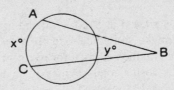

(A) ½y

(B) y

(C) ½x

(D) ½ (x − y)

29. What is the value of sec 45°?

(A) $\dfrac{\sqrt{2}}{2}$

(B) $\sqrt{2}$

(C) $\sqrt{3}$

(D) 2

30. If $(a - b)^2 = 40$ and $ab = 8$, find $a^2 + b^2$.

(A) 5

(B) 24

(C) 48

(D) 56

31. What is $\frac{1}{5}$% of 40?

(A) 8

(B) .8

(C) .08

(D) .008

32. In right triangle ABC below, what is the value of tan B?

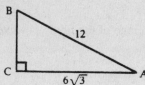

(A) $\frac{1}{2}$

(B) $\dfrac{\sqrt{2}}{2}$

(C) 1

(D) $\sqrt{3}$

33. A television set listed at $160 is offered at a $12\frac{1}{2}$% discount during a storewide sale. If an additional 3% is allowed on the net price for payment in cash, how much is Josh's total savings if he buys this set during the sale for cash?

(A) $24.36

(B) $24.80

(C) $17.20

(D) $24.20

34. The square root of 17,689 is exactly

(A) 131

(B) 132

(C) 133

(D) 134

35. On consecutive days, the high temperature in Great Neck was 86°, 82°, 90°, 92°, 80°, and 81°. What was the high temperature on the seventh day, if the average high for the week was 84°?

(A) 79°

(B) 85°

(C) 81°

(D) 77°

36. 80 is $12\frac{1}{2}$% of what number?

(A) 10

(B) 100

(C) 64

(D) 640

37. A flagpole casts a shadow of 27 feet when the sun is 30° above the horizon. How many feet high is the flagpole?

(A) 13

(B) $9\sqrt{2}$

(C) $9\sqrt{3}$

(D) 27

38. Solve for a: $8 - 4(a - 1) = 2 + 3(4 - a)$

(A) $-\frac{5}{3}$

(B) $-\frac{7}{3}$

(C) 2

(D) -2

39. A farmer uses 140 feet of fencing to enclose a rectangular field. If the ratio of length to width is 3:4, find the diagonal, in feet, of the field.

(A) 50

(B) 100

(C) 20

(D) 10

40. 4 is what percent of 80?

(A) 20

(B) 2

(C) 5

(D) .5

41. Solve for y: 2x + 3y = 12b
3x − y = 7b

(A) $7\frac{1}{7}$b

(B) 2b

(C) 3b

(D) $1\frac{2}{7}$

42. Find the number of degrees in the sum of the interior angles of a hexagon.

(A) 360

(B) 540

(C) 720

(D) 900

43. Solve for x: $x^2 − 8x − 20 = 0$

(A) 5 or −4

(B) 10 or −2

(C) −5 or 4

(D) −10 or −2

44. 36 is 150% of what number?

(A) 24

(B) 54

(C) 26

(D) 12

45. Marie has $2.20 in dimes and quarters. If the number of dimes is ¼ the number of quarters, how many dimes doe she have?

(A) 2

(B) 4

(C) 6

(D) 8

46. A balloon is fastened to a cable which makes an angle of 60° with the horizontal. If 300 feet of cable is let out, how high, in feet, is the balloon?

(A) 150

(B) $150\sqrt{2}$

(C) $150\sqrt{3}$

(D) $300\sqrt{2}$

47. Mark is now 4 times as old as his brother Stephen. In 1 year Mark will be 3 times as old as Stephen will be then. How old was Mark two years ago?

(A) 2

(B) 3

(C) 6

(D) 8

48. In driving from San Francisco to Los Angeles, Arthur drove for three hours at 60 miles per hour and for 4 hours at 55 miles per hour. What was his average rate, in miles per hour, for the entire trip?

(A) 57.5

(B) 56.9

(C) 57.1

(D) 58.2

49. If the length and width of a rectangle are each doubled, the area is increased by

(A) 50%

(B) 100%

(C) 200%

(D) 300%

50. A ball rolls down a ramp which makes an angle of 45° with the horizontal. When the ball rolls 40 inches along the ramp, how many inches has the ball moved in the vertical direction?

(A) 20

(B) $20\sqrt{2}$

(C) $20\sqrt{3}$

(D) 40

End of Quantitative Ability Section

If you finish your work on this Quantitative Ability section before time is called, check your work on this section only. Do not return to the Verbal Ability Section. Do not go on to the next section until the signal is given.

BIOLOGY

50 questions

Directions: Choose the best answer to each question and mark its letter on your answer sheet.

1. In a population the frequency of the N allele is .8 and the frequency of the n allele is .2. The proportion of offspring that contain the n allele is

   (A) 4%.

   (B) 32%.

   (C) 36%.

   (D) 64%.

2. All chordates possess

   (A) vertebrae.

   (B) cryptic coloration.

   (C) a notochord.

   (D) the chorda tympanum.

3. Bryophytes

   (A) usually lack vascular tissue.

   (B) usually lack a dominant haploid gametophyte stage.

   (C) include club mosses and horsetails.

   (D) do not require water for fertilization.

4. The type of muscle tissue found within the walls of blood vessels and of other internal organs in humans is

   (A) striated muscle.

   (B) skeletal muscle.

   (C) voluntary muscle.

   (D) smooth muscle.

5. Which of the following is a saprophyte?

   (A) shark

   (B) mushroom

   (C) fern

   (D) ponderosa pine

6. Most absorption of digestive products in humans occurs in the

   (A) stomach.

   (B) small intestine.

   (C) large intestine.

   (D) pancreas.

7. Polypeptide chains are synthesized in the

   (A) golgi apparatus.

   (B) nucleus.

   (C) lysosomes.

   (D) ribosomes.

8. RNA genes are found only in some

   (A) viruses.

   (B) cyanobacteria.

   (C) blue-green algae.

   (D) horseshoe crabs.

9. Bacteria

   (A) are never photosynthetic.

   (B) use mitochondria for respiration.

   (C) use ATP to synthesize complex organic compounds.

   (D) reproduce through fusion.

10. White blood cell count can be used to determine whether a patient has

(A) diabetes.

(B) the Rh factor.

(C) an infection.

(D) hormonal problems.

11. The part of the human eye that contains rod and cone cells is the

(A) iris.

(B) lens.

(C) choroid.

(D) retina.

12. At the end of mitotic cell division in eucaryotes

(A) four new haploid cells result.

(B) two new haploid cells result.

(C) four new diploid cells result.

(D) two new diploid cells result.

13. Crossing over occurs during

(A) prophase of mitosis.

(B) anaphase of mitosis.

(C) first prophase of meiosis.

(D) first anaphase of meiosis.

14. During which process would there be a net movement of glucose molecules through a membrane from a region of lower concentration to a region of higher concentration?

(A) passive transport

(B) active transport

(C) osmosis

(D) heterosis

15. A somatic cell of a person with Down's syndrome will have how many chromosomes?

(A) 23

(B) 24

(C) 46

(D) 47

16. Color blindness is a recessive sex-linked trait in humans. If a color-blind male mates with a non–color-blind female homozygous for the trait, what is the chance that their daughter will be color blind?

(A) 0%

(B) 25%

(C) 50%

(D) 100%

17. Deoxygenated blood enters the right atrium of the human heart. Choose the correct pathway for the blood after it leaves the right atrium:

(A) right ventricle—aorta—pulmonary veins—pulmonary artery—left ventricle—left atrium

(B) pulmonary veins—pulmonary artery—right ventricle—left ventricle—left atrium—aorta

(C) right ventricle—pulmonary artery—pulmonary veins—left atrium—left ventricle—aorta

(D) right ventricle—pulmonary artery—pulmonary veins—aorta—left atrium—left ventricle

18. Which of the following is NOT a direct requirement for photosynthesis to occur in most plants?

(A) carbon dioxide

(B) chlorophyll

(C) ADP

(D) glucose

19. Which of the following is not an RNA nucleotide base?

(A) adenine

(B) guanine

(C) cytosine

(D) thymine

20. Which of the following is NOT true of messenger RNA?

(A) mRNA carries amino acids to the ribosomes during protein synthesis.

(B) mRNA is produced from nuclear DNA during transcription.

(C) mRNA carries information from the nucleus to the ribosomes specifying protein amino acid sequences.

(D) mRNA is mostly composed of long segments of codons that will not be translated into proteins.

21. During aerobic respiration, oxygen

(A) changes proteins to amino acids.

(B) aids in glucose formation.

(C) aids in pyruvic acid formation.

(D) acts as the final acceptor of hydrogen.

22. Bean plants bearing homozygous wrinkled seeds are crossed with bean plants bearing homozygous smooth seeds. All of the offspring bear smooth seeds. This illustrates the principle of

(A) incomplete dominance.

(B) dominance.

(C) independent assortment

(D) segregation.

23. Which of the following enhances propagation of a nerve impulse along a nerve fiber?

(A) nonmyelinated nerve fibers

(B) excess sodium inside the nerve fibers

(C) polarization of the nerve cell so that inside is negative relative to outside

(D) increased diameter of nerve fibers

24. Which of the following would normally work against the process of speciation?

(A) allopatric populations

(B) sympatric populations

(C) founder effect and genetic drift

(D) populations living in different microclimates

25. Mammals are distinguished from all other vertebrates in that

(A) only mammals bear live young.

(B) only mammals are endothermic.

(C) only mammals have completely four-chambered hearts.

(D) only mammals have three bones in the middle ear.

26. During development, the archenteron

(A) will form the cavity of the digestive tract.

(B) will become the anus.

(C) is part of the blastula.

(D) forms right above the neural groove.

27. An organic catalyst that lowers the activation energy required for biological reactions is called

(A) a carotenoid.

(B) a lipid.

(C) an enzyme

(D) a hormone.

28. When a living cell is placed in a medium that is hypertonic relative to it

(A) the cell will shrink.

(B) the cell will expand.

(C) the cell will either shrink or expand depending on temperature.

(D) the cell will either shrink or expand depending on the sodium-potassium gradient.

29. A person whose T cells are not functioning properly

(A) will suffer from a thyroid imbalance.

(B) will have impaired immune response to foreign substances.

(C) will not be able to digest sugars.

(D) will have impaired renal function.

30. Which of the following has NOT been an adaptation of plants to life on land?

(A) pollen

(B) large, independent sporophyte

(C) seeds

(D) pronounced haploid phase

31. In which structure of a plant would a developing seed be found?

(A) pollen

(B) anther

(C) stigma

(D) ovary

32. Of the following, the structure that undergoes the LEAST amount of change during mitosis is the
    (A) mitochondria.
    (B) nucleus.
    (C) centriole.
    (D) ribosomes.

33. An organism with a hard exoskeleton, five pairs of jointed legs, and filter-feeding apparatus is
    (A) a tunicate.
    (B) a crustacean.
    (C) an insect.
    (D) an echinoderm.

34. Which cell part contains no DNA?
    (A) mitochondrion
    (B) cell vacuole
    (C) spindle fiber
    (D) nucleolus

35. Rapid repeated mitotic division of a fertilized egg is called
    (A) gametogenesis.
    (B) cleavage.
    (C) neurulation.
    (D) reduction division.

36. Follicles in the human female are stimulated by a hormone secreted by the
    (A) pituitary gland.
    (B) adrenal gland.
    (C) uterus.
    (D) ovary.

37. A girl has brown hair and brown eyes and her sister has brown hair and blue eyes. Their different combinations of traits are best explained by
    (A) independent assortment.
    (B) incomplete dominance.
    (C) sex linkage.
    (D) multiple alleles.

38. Which is the correct pathway for cellular formation and secretion of enzymes?
    (A) nuclear DNA—mRNA—ribosome—golgi apparatus—lysosome—cytosol
    (B) nuclear DNA—mRNA—endoplasmic reticulum—lysosome—golgi apparatus—cytosol
    (C) nuclear DNA—mRNA—golgi apparatus—endoplasmic reticulum—ribosome—cytosol
    (D) nuclear DNA—mRNA—lysosome—golgi apparatus—endoplasmic reticulum—ribosome—cytosol

39. Wrinkled green seeds (RRGG) are crossed with round yellow seeds (rrgg). Wrinkled is dominant over round and green is dominant over yellow. What will the phenotype of seeds in the F_1 generation be?
    (A) All will be wrinkled and green.
    (B) All will have some intermediate phenotype between wrinkled green and round yellow.
    (C) There will be a mixture of wrinkled green, wrinkled yellow, smooth green, and smooth yellow.
    (D) There will be a 3:1 ratio of wrinkled green : smooth yellow seeds.

40. In the above question, if the F_1 progeny are randomly mated, what will the phenotype of seeds in the F_2 generation be?
    (A) All will be wrinkled and green.
    (B) All will have some intermediate phenotype between wrinkled green and smooth yellow.
    (C) There will be a ratio of 9 wrinkled green : 3 wrinkled yellow : 3 smooth green : 1 smooth yellow.
    (D) There will be a 3:1 ratio of wrinkled green: smooth yellow seeds.

41. The limbic system of the human brain
    (A) processes most complex sensory information.
    (B) controls feelings and emotions.
    (C) is the control center or "relay station" for the brain.
    (D) processes visual and audio information.

42. In human beings, the ulna is found

    (A) at the forefront of the cerebral cortex.

    (B) at the juncture between the left ventricle and the aorta.

    (C) in the stomach lining.

    (D) in the forearm.

43. Which of the following is NOT a requirement of the Hardy-Weinberg Law?

    (A) Mating must be completely random with respect to genotype.

    (B) Reproductive success must be completely based on adaptive advantages of some genotypes over others.

    (C) Mutations must not occur.

    (D) Populations must be large enough to avoid genetic drift.

44. Which factor has the largest effect on the rate of evolution of organisms?

    (A) use and disuse

    (B) binary fission

    (C) vegetative propagation

    (D) environmental fluxes

45. Which equation represents a process in animals that releases the greatest amount of energy per molecule of substrate?

    (A) glucose ▶ ethyl alcohol + carbon dioxide + energy

    (B) hydrogen + carbon dioxide ▶ PGAL (phosphoglyceraldehyde)

    (C) water + chlorophyll + light ▶ hydrogen + oxygen

    (D) glucose + oxygen ▶ water + carbon dioxide + energy

46. Which is NOT an endocrine gland?

    (A) gall bladder

    (B) testis

    (C) thyroid

    (D) pancreas

47. The arm of a human, the wing of a bird, and the flipper of a dolphin are

    (A) analogous structures.

    (B) examples of convergent evolution.

    (C) homologous structures.

    (D) related only in that they have similar functions.

48. Toxic products of plant metabolism are stored in the

    (A) chloroplasts.

    (B) vacuoles.

    (C) stomata.

    (D) basal bodies.

49. Glycogen is most similar in structure and composition to

    (A) glycerol.

    (B) potato starch.

    (C) leukocytes.

    (D) nitrogenous wastes.

50. A family has four girls and one boy. What is the chance that the next child will be a boy?

    (A) 20%

    (B) 25%

    (C) 50%

    (D) 80%

End of Biology Section

If you finish your work on this section before time is called, check your work on this section only. Do not return to either previous section. Do not go on to the next section until the signal is given.

CHEMISTRY

50 questions

Directions: Choose the best answer to each question and mark its letter on your answer sheet.

1. An atom's mass number is equal to the total number of its

    (A) electrons only.

    (B) electrons and protons.

    (C) protons and neutrons.

    (D) electrons, protons, and neutrons.

2. Which of the following is NOT a postulate of Dalton's Atomic Theory?

    (A) Atoms compose all matter and can neither be destroyed nor created.

    (B) Atoms of a given element are identical in size, mass, and shape.

    (C) Chemical reactions occur when atoms unite or separate.

    (D) Atoms concentrate mass and positive charge in their nuclei.

3. What is the total number of electrons in the 2p sublevel of a sulfur atom (atomic number = 16)?

    (A) 6

    (B) 2

    (C) 3

    (D) 5

4. Which electron configuration represents an atom in an excited state?

    (A) $1s^2 2s^2$

    (B) $1s^2 2s^2 2p^1$

    (C) $1s^2 2s^2 2p^5$

    (D) $1s^2 2s^2 2p^5 3s^1$

5. Which of the following have no known stable isotopes?

    (A) the halogens

    (B) the inert gases

    (C) elements with an atomic number less than 10

    (D) elements with an atomic number greater than 83

6. Emission of energy will accompany which electron transmission?

    (A) 1s to 2s

    (B) 2p to 3s

    (C) 3p to 3s

    (D) 3s to 3p

7. In the compound $C_6H_{12}O_6$, for every one atom of carbon, how many atoms of hydrogen are there?

    (A) 1

    (B) ½

    (C) 2

    (D) 12

8. In the compound $C_6H_{12}O_6$, for every one mole of carbon, how many moles of hydrogen are there?

    (A) 1

    (B) ½

    (C) 2

    (D) 12

9. What is the mass in grams of 4 atoms of CO_2?

    (A) 22

    (B) 44

    (C) 88

    (D) 176

10. A 1-mole sample of helium is at STP. If the temperature remains constant and the pressure is halved, the new volume will be
    (A) 11.2 liters.
    (B) 22.4 liters.
    (C) 33.6 liters.
    (D) 44.8 liters.

11. When the equation $H_2 + Fe_3O_2 \blacktriangleright Fe + H_2O$ is completely balanced using smallest whole numbers, the coefficient of H_2 is
    (A) 1.
    (B) 2.
    (C) 3.
    (D) 4.

12. The percent by mass of sodium in NaC1 (formula mass = 56) is closest to
    (A) 10%.
    (B) 40%.
    (C) 65%.
    (D) 80%.

13. How many molecules are in one mole of sodium?
    (A) 1×10^{23}
    (B) 6×10^{23}
    (C) 11×10^{23}
    (D) 12.9×10^{23}

14. Formation of an ionic bond would be likely between
    (A) Mg and C1.
    (B) Mg and He.
    (C) Mg and Ca.
    (D) Mg and H.

15. When hydrogen bonds to oxygen, energy is
    (A) always released.
    (B) always absorbed.
    (C) neither absorbed nor released.
    (D) either absorbed or released depending on initial molecular state.

16. When two atoms of C1 combine to make $C1_2$, which of the following is NOT true?
    (A) Electrons are shared between the two atoms.
    (B) There will be van der Waals forces between the two atoms.
    (C) The atoms will form an ionic bond.
    (D) Energy will be released.

17. Hydrogen bonds are strongest between molecules of
    (A) HF.
    (B) HC1.
    (C) HBr.
    (D) HI.

18. Of the following, the element with the lowest electronegativity is
    (A) C1.
    (B) K.
    (C) H.
    (D) O.

19. The majority of the elements in the periodic table are
    (A) gases.
    (B) metals.
    (C) halogens.
    (D) metalloids.

20. Which element is a liquid at STP?
    (A) I
    (B) Se
    (C) Li
    (D) Hg

21. Of the following, the most active metal is
    (A) Na.
    (B) A1.
    (C) Fe.
    (D) Sn.

22. Of the following, the one most likely to be a poor conductor of heat and electricity and to bond with other elements to make acidic compounds is

    (A) C1.

    (B) Mg.

    (C) Zn.

    (D) Li.

23. How many calories of heat are needed to raise 100 g of water by 5 degrees?

    (A) .05 calories

    (B) 20 calories

    (C) 500 calories

    (D) 5000 calories

24. Which is an example of an endothermic phase change?

    (A) liquid to gas

    (B) gas to liquid

    (C) liquid to solid

    (D) gas to liquid

25. When heat energy is lost by a pure liquid at its vaporization point, its potential energy

    (A) decreases.

    (B) increases.

    (C) stays the same.

    (D) initially decreases, then increases

26. A container of helium has a volume of 100 ml at STP. What will be the new volume of the helium if temperature remains the same and pressure is increased to 1140 torr?

    (A) 10 ml

    (B) 150 ml

    (C) 66.7 ml

    (D) 667 ml

27. When a substance undergoes sublimation it

    (A) loses potential energy at its freezing point.

    (B) liquefies.

    (C) solidifies.

    (D) changes from a solid directly to a gas.

28. Litmus paper exposed to hydrochloric acid will

    (A) turn red.

    (B) turn blue.

    (C) not change color.

    (D) turn red or blue, depending on temperature.

29. When water is electrolyzed, which of the following are the products obtained?

    (A) H^+ and OH^-

    (B) H_2 and OH

    (C) H_2 and O_2

    (D) H_2O_2

30. The pH of a solution whose H_3O^+ is 0.001 mole per liter is

    (A) acidic.

    (B) basic.

    (C) neutral.

    (D) alkaline.

31. Which of the following statements best distinguishes electrolytes from non-electrolytes?

    (A) Electrolytes are usually covalent compounds while non-electrolytes are usually ionic compounds.

    (B) Electrolytes are always ionic compounds while non-electrolytes are always covalent compounds.

    (C) Non-electrolytes are usually insoluble in water while electrolytes are usually soluble.

    (D) Electrolytes can be covalent or ionic compounds but must be ionic in solution.

32. If the [OH⁻] = 1 × 10⁻² at 298 for a given solution, the [H⁺] of the solution is equal to

   (A) 1×10^{-2}.

   (B) 1×10^{-5}.

   (C) 1×10^{-9}.

   (D) 1×10^{-12}.

33. What could be the pH of a solution whose OH⁻ ion concentration is less than its H_3O^+ concentration?

   (A) 3

   (B) 7

   (C) 9

   (D) 14

34. The correctly balanced half-reaction for the reduction of Al^{3+} to Al is

   (A) $Al^{3+} \rightarrow 3Al + 3e^-$.

   (B) $Al^{3+} + 3e^- \rightarrow Al$.

   (C) $Al^{3+} \rightarrow Al + 3e^-$.

   (D) $Al^{3+} + 3e^- \rightarrow 3Al$.

35. For a neutral molecule of H_2O

   (A) the oxidation number of hydrogen is 1+ and the oxidation number of oxygen is 2−.

   (B) the oxidation number of hydrogen is 2− and the oxidation number of oxygen is 1+.

   (C) the oxidation number of hydrogen is 2+ and the oxidation number of oxygen is 2−.

   (D) the oxidation number of hydrogen is 1− and the oxidation number of oxygen is 1+.

36. In the reaction $2Na + Cl_2 \rightarrow 2 NaCl$

   (A) chlorine is the oxidizing agent and sodium is the reducing agent.

   (B) sodium is the oxidizing agent and chlorine is the reducing agent.

   (C) chlorine is being oxidized and sodium is being reduced.

   (D) chlorine is supplying electrons and sodium is picking up electrons.

37. Which change in oxidation number represents reduction?

   (A) −2 to −1

   (B) +2 to +3

   (C) 0 to −1

   (D) −1 to +1

38. Catalysts

   (A) alter the ratio of products of a reaction.

   (B) alter the rate of reactions.

   (C) alter both the ratio of products and rate of reactions.

   (D) alter neither the ratio of products nor the rate of reactions.

39. Which of the following will NOT generally speed up the rate of a reaction?

   (A) increasing the temperature

   (B) adding a catalyst

   (C) increasing the concentration of reactants

   (D) decreasing the air pressure

40. When a solid sublimates, the entropy of the system

   (A) increases.

   (B) decreases.

   (C) remains the same.

   (D) may increase or decrease.

41. Which equilibrium constant indicates an equilibrium mixture that most favors formation of products?

   (A) $K_{eg} = 1 \times 10^{-5}$

   (B) $K_{eg} = 1 \times 10^{0}$

   (C) $K_{eg} = 1 \times 10^{1}$

   (D) $K_{eg} = 1 \times 10^{4}$

42. The isotope $_6C^{14}$ has

(A) 6 carbons.

(B) 8 protons.

(C) 20 atoms.

(D) 6 electrons.

43. Isotopes of a given element have

(A) the same number of protons and electrons.

(B) the same number of neutrons but different numbers of electrons.

(C) the same atomic number but different atomic weights.

(D) different atomic numbers but the same atomic weights.

44. At the end of one hour, ¼ of an original sample of a radioactive element remains. What is the half-life of the element?

(A) 15 minutes

(B) 30 minutes

(C) 4 hours

(D) 16 hours

45. Which of the following is an alcohol?

(A) CH_3CH_2OH

(B) CH_4

(C) $C_6H_{12}O_6$

(D) $CH_3CH_2NH_2$

46. CH_3COH is

(A) an aldehyde.

(B) an ester.

(C) a ketone.

(D) an amine.

47. Which formula represents a saturated hydrocarbon?

(A) CH_4

(B) C_4H_{10}

(C) C_4H_6

(D) C_4H_2

48. Alcohols react with organic acids to form

(A) aldehydes.

(B) esters.

(C) ketones.

(D) amines.

49. Which of the following has the lowest boiling point?

(A) methane

(B) propane

(C) butane

(D) octane

50. Ethyl alcohol is the product of which kind of reaction?

(A) saponification

(B) fermentation

(C) esterification

(D) redox-elimination

End of Chemistry Section

If you finish your work on this section before time is called, check your work on this section only. Do not return to any previous section. Do not go on to the next section until the signal is given.

READING COMPREHENSION

45 questions

Directions: Read each passage and answer the questions following it.

Passage for questions 1 to 5:

The function of the heart is to discharge, with adequate force, an amount of blood sufficient for the metabolic needs of the body. The amount discharged in a unit of time is determined by the stroke, volume, and rate of heartbeat. As the demand for blood by the body varies from moment to moment, it is evident that the rate, force, and systolic output of the heart must be governed in accordance. This control is both neural and humoral.

The origin of the heartbeat is not dependent upon the central nervous system. But it is a fact, proved by everyday observation, that the state of mind or body can modify the action of the heart. The heart is connected with the central nervous system by means of two nerves, the vagus and the cervical sympathetic. From the brain there issue twelve pairs of cranial nerves; of these the vagus, or pneumogastric nerve, forms the tenth pair. The vagus springs from the lowest division of the brain, known as the medulla oblongata, which may be looked upon as the connection between the brain and the spinal cord. This nerve is very widely distributed, sending branches to the heart, lungs, trachea, esophagus, stomach, pancreas, gall bladder, intestines, etc.; it is, therefore, one of the most important nerves in the body. To the heart the vagus nerve sends both afferent and efferent fibers; the latter fibers belong to the autonomic nervous system. The efferent vagal fibers end in a peripheral ganglion lying in the heart; from this ganglion the impulses are carried by very short postganglionic fibers to the sinoauricular and the auriculoventricular nodes and the bundle of His.

1. The statement that the vagus nerve is connected with involuntary action is

    (A) contrary to the paragraphs.

    (B) neither made nor implied in the paragraphs.

    (C) definitely stated by the author.

    (D) not made, but implied in the paragraphs.

2. Which of the following statements is *least* true of the vagus nerve? The vagus nerve

    (A) becomes the autonomic system.

    (B) comes from the medulla oblongata.

    (C) is one of the tenth pair of cranial nerves.

    (D) serves the heart through both efferent and afferent fibers.

3. Which of the phrases makes the following statement most nearly true? "The rate, force and systolic output of the heart are controlled by —————."

    (A) neural connections

    (B) the sinoauricular node

    (C) the bundle of His

    (D) the vagus and cervical sympathetic systems

4. That the state of mind can modify heart action is

    (A) shown to operate through the vagus nerve.

    (B) shown to operate through control from the brain.

    (C) shown by cardiac inhibition.

    (D) stated, but its mode of operation is not shown.

5. The function of the heart is to

    (A) clear impurities from the blood.

    (B) pump blood throughout the body.

    (C) regulate the emotions.

    (D) stimulate the vagus nerve.

Passage for questions 6 to 10:

A colored transparent object, such as a piece of red glass, transmits red light and absorbs all or most of the other colors that shine on it. But what about opaque (nontransparent) objects? Why is one piece of cloth red, for example, while another is blue? The answer is that we see only the light that is reflected from such an object. White light, which contains all colors, shines on our piece of cloth. The dye in the cloth is of such a nature that it pretty well absorbs all colors except red. The red is then reflected, and that is what we see. If some other color or combination of colors is reflected, then we may get any hue or tint. Incidentally, this gives us a hint as to why many fabrics seem to have one color under artificial light and another color in daylight. The artificial light is of a different composition from daylight, and therefore the amount of each color reflected is different.

Light from an incandescent lamp, for example, contains proportionately more red and yellow than does sunlight, and hence emphasizes the red and yellow hues, weakening the blues and violets by contrast. Strangely enough, though, yellow may appear quite white under an incandescent lamp. This comes about because our eyes, being accustomed to the yellowish light from the lamp, no longer distinguish the lamplight from the real white of sunlight. Therefore, a piece of yellow cloth or paper, reflecting all the colors contained in the lamplight, appears to be white.

6. If an object were manufactured so that all light rays that hit it were reflected away from it, the color of the object would be

(A) white.

(B) black.

(C) iridescent.

(D) transparent.

7. If an object absorbed all the light that strikes it, the color of the object would be

(A) white.

(B) black.

(C) iridescent.

(D) transparent.

8. If an object were made in such a way that the light striking it was neither reflected nor absorbed, the object would be

(A) white.

(B) black.

(C) translucent.

(D) transparent

9. If the light from a blue mercury lamp which contains no red light waves were to illuminate a pure red tie, the tie would appear to be

(A) white.

(B) black.

(C) red.

(D) transparent.

10. Artificial light

I. is different from sunlight.

II. contains more red and yellow than sunlight.

III. appears more like sunlight with a green shade.

IV. makes glass transparent.

(A) I only

(B) I and II

(C) I, II, and III

(D) I, II, III, and IV

Passage for questions 11 to 15:

Over the last few decades, medical knowledge has advanced at a phenomenal rate. Physicians now understand structures and processes which only 40 or even 30 years ago they did not even know existed. We can reasonably expect that the ability to manipulate and change these structures and processes will soon follow.

One of the most fascinating and promising—yet frightening—areas of medical advancement is DNA technology. DNA stands for deoxyribonucleic acid. DNA is a component of genetic material. Scientists have found that by recombining DNA they can actually change an animal's genetic makeup. Genetic researchers have tampered with DNA and have produced a strain of "supermouse." These supermice are more than twice the size of normal mice of their species. Genetically superior cattle have been bred through isolation of superior genes.

Medically the prospects are very exciting. Researchers are not yet ready to predict a target date, but probably within our lifetime they will be able to "repair" defective human genes. The technology is already in place for identifying a fetus which will be born with a genetic disease. Embryology is not quite so far advanced, but we can envision that in the future the genes of a hemophiliac embryo may be repaired so that the baby will not be born a hemophiliac. Or perhaps the embryo which was genetically programmed to inherit hypertension can be spared this affliction through genetic repair. Another possibility is that genetic manipulation will be accomplished even before fertilization. There are still many unknown factors, but there is real hope for eventual eradication of genetic diseases.

Along with the useful potential of genetic engineering comes the frightening prospect of its misuse. Unscrupulous researchers might experiment with humans and create "Frankenstein's monsters." And unanswered questions arise: When the ability to do so arrives, should we breed genetic "supermen"? Should we even try to create genetically altered human beings? Should we breed a lower species of human being to do distasteful work? If we choose to predetermine the heredity of humans and to breed "to order," who has the right to choose which shall be super-intelligent and which only marginally functional?

A presidential commission is urging that guidelines be set now to determine how genetic material should be influenced in the future. The subject of bioethics is being discussed within clerical, scientific, and political circles and has even become a cocktail party conversation topic.

11. DNA is

   (A) the cause of hemophilia.

   (B) a scientific organization.

   (C) a component of genes.

   (D) a presidential commission.

12. The question "Should genetic screening for health defects be used as a basis for job selection?" is

   (A) a medical question.

   (B) a bioethical question.

   (C) a business question.

   (D) a religious question.

13. The term *bioengineering* refers to

   (A) the coaching of marathon runners.

   (B) the use of artificial limbs.

   (C) organic animal husbandry.

   (D) manipulating genetic material.

14. According to the passage, the application of the new genetic technology to disease control is

   (A) possible.

   (B) unlikely.

   (C) already in progress.

   (D) predicted to occur within ten years.

15. The moral and ethical ramifications of our ability to alter human beings are of concern to

   (A) the President.

   (B) Congress.

   (C) members of the clergy.

   (D) all of us.

Passage for questions 16 to 20:

There is evidence that the usual variety of high blood pressure is, in part, a familial disease. Since families have similar genes as well as similar environments, familial diseases could be due to shared genetic influences, to shared environmental factors, or to both. For some years, the role of one environmental factor commonly shared by families, namely dietary salt (i.e., sodium chloride), has been studied at Brookhaven National Laboratory. These studies suggest that chronic excess salt ingestion can lead to high blood pressure in man and animals. Some individuals, however, and some rats consume large amounts of salt without developing high blood pressure. No matter how strictly all environmental factors were controlled in these experiments, some salt-fed animals never developed hypertension whereas a few rapidly developed very severe hypertension followed by early death. These marked variations were interpreted to result from differences in genetic constitution.

By mating in successive generations only those animals that failed to develop hypertension from salt ingestion, a resistant strain (the ''R'' strain) has been evolved in which consumption of large quantities of salt fails to influence the blood pressure significantly. In contrast, by mating only animals that quickly develop hypertension from salt, a sensitive strain (''S'' strain) has also been developed.

The availability of these two strains permits investigations not heretofore possible. They provide a plausible laboratory model on which to investigate some clinical aspects of the human prototypes of hypertension. More important, there might be the possibility of developing methods by which genetic susceptibility of human beings to high blood pressure can be defined without waiting for its appearance. Radioactive sodium 22 was an important ''tool'' in working out the characteristics of the sodium chloride metabolism.

16. The statement that best relates to the main idea of this article is:

   (A) When salt is added to their diets, rats and humans react in much the same way.

   (B) The near future will see a cure for high blood pressure.

   (C) Modern research has shown that high blood pressure is a result of salt in the diet.

   (D) A tendency toward high blood pressure may be a hereditary factor.

17. The study of the effects of salt on high blood pressure was carried out

   (A) because members of the same family tend to use similar amounts of salt.

   (B) to explore the long-term use of a sodium-based substance.

   (C) because it was proven that salt caused high blood pressure.

   (D) because of the availability of chemically pure salt and its derivatives.

18. It can be implied that the main difference between ''S'' and ''R'' rats is their

   (A) need for sodium 22.

   (B) rate of mating.

   (C) reaction to salt.

   (D) type of blood.

19. The reader can infer from the article that sodium 22 can be used to

   (A) cure high blood pressure caused by salt.

   (B) tell the ''S'' rats from the ''R'' rats.

   (C) determine what a sodium chloride metabolism is like.

   (D) control high blood pressure.

20. Among the results of the research discussed in this article, the most beneficial might be

   (A) the early identification of potential high blood pressure victims.

   (B) development of diets free of salt.

   (C) an early cure for high blood pressure.

   (D) control of genetic agents that cause high blood pressure.

Passage for questions 21 to 25:

One of the most important experiments in photosynthesis was performed by the English scientist Joseph Priestley. Priestley believed that mint could restore oxygen to an atmosphere from which this gas had been removed. To test this he placed a burning candle in a closed jar. Quickly the flame went out. A mouse was then placed in the jar; it, too, quickly died. From this Priestley concluded that a burning candle and a living mouse both extracted the same substance from the air. Priestley observed by chance that a sprig of mint had the effect of restoring the injured air to a normal state. A mouse now placed in the jar thrived as though it were breathing atmospheric air.

The experiment made by Priestley was soon followed by others. Other plants besides mint were tested and were found to have the same effect on the atmosphere as mint. It was later found that it was only the green parts of plants that possessed the ability to produce oxygen. Moreover, it was found that the formation of oxygen occurred only in the presence of sunlight. It was further shown that in the process of adding oxygen to the air, plants simultaneously extracted another gaseous material, a substance we now know as carbon dioxide. In addition to the exchange of gases with the surrounding air there was the growth of the plant itself. From the above it was confirmed that plants consumed carbon dioxide in the production of organic material and oxygen. The plant gained considerable weight during the process. It was later established that the overall gain in weight, together with the weight of oxygen given off, equaled the weight of all the raw materials consumed by the plant. These raw materials consisted partly of the carbon dioxide removed from the air but largely of water, incorporated by the plant through a number of complex chemical processes.

21. If in Priestley's experiment the sprig of mint had been replaced by blades of grass, the results would most likely have been

    (A) inconclusive.

    (B) similar.

    (C) different.

    (D) unchanged.

22. "Priestley believed that mint could restore oxygen to an atmosphere from which the gas had been removed" can best be described as a statement of a(n)

    (A) observation.

    (B) conclusion.

    (C) hypothesis.

    (D) analysis.

23. According to this passage, which of the following would contain the greatest concentration of oxygen?

    (A) desert land

    (B) cave

    (C) wheat field

    (D) ice field

24. We may infer from reading this passage that plants produce oxygen

    (A) independently of sunlight.

    (B) only in the presence of sunlight.

    (C) at any time of day.

    (D) in their brown stems.

25. Which of the following statements is most essential for the conclusion that "plants consume carbon dioxide in photosynthesis"?

    (A) Plants extracted another gaseous material.

    (B) Only the green parts of plants produce oxygen.

    (C) Mint restored the injured air.

    (D) The plant gained considerable weight.

Passage for questions 26 to 30:

Dr. Horace O. Parrack of the United States Air Force Medical Laboratory has been studying the effect on airmen of jet propulsion and other modern aircraft engines. The Army wants to know whether or not high-pitched sounds generated by the new power planes are hazardous. Jet-engine noise may temporarily deafen a man even after brief exposures, and repeated exposure may result in permanent deafness.

Dr. Parrack finds that rats and guinea pigs can be killed with high-frequency sound waves, but that man is safe against them because he has no fur. With the fur-bearing animals the sound energy is turned into heat. They die from high-frequency noise because they get so hot that the body proteins coagulate. When the hair is shaved off, there is no such coagulating effect. Man, with his much more efficient skin ventilating system, is safe at energy levels 120 times greater than rats are.

26. The ultimate purpose of Dr. Parrack's study is

    (A) to suggest safer flying methods.

    (B) to reduce loss of life in animals.

    (C) to study causes of deafness.

    (D) to decrease danger to aviators who fly jet-propelled planes.

27. According to this study

    (A) high-pitched sounds are not at all dangerous.

    (B) high-pitched sounds can be fatal to man.

    (C) high-pitched sounds often cause deafness.

    (D) high-pitched sounds decrease body heat.

28. Animals like rats and guinea pigs may be killed by high-frequency sounds because

    (A) their blood gets too hot.

    (B) their fur does not allow body heat to escape.

    (C) they are fed on proteins.

    (D) their blood coagulates.

29. Coagulation means most nearly

    (A) thinning out.

    (B) clotting.

    (C) boiling.

    (D) burning.

30. The efficient ventilating system that man has includes

    (A) intestines.

    (B) throat.

    (C) skin pores.

    (D) mouth.

Passage for questions 31 to 34:

The genetic material is now known to be deoxyribonucleic acid (DNA). The two general functions of DNA are (1) replication for the propagation of life, and (2) serving as a template for protein synthesis. It is this second function that we shall outline here. The initial step is the assemblage of messenger ribonucleic acid (mRNA) by DNA. This process is known as transcription. The mRNA then acts as a complement of the genetic code in the DNA molecule that assembled it. The mRNA then directs the assembly of a protein from an available pool of protein building blocks, amino acids. This process is known as translation. Therefore, we can summarize protein synthesis as transcription and translation. A second kind of RNA, known as transfer ribonucleic acid (tRNA), is responsible for directing the correct amino acid to its correct place in the amino acid sequence that is to become the protein.

31. The title that best expresses the content of this passage is

    (A) The Mechanism of Protein Synthesis.

    (B) The Structure and Function of DNA.

    (C) Sexual and Asexual Reproduction.

    (D) The Chemistry of Life.

32. According to the passage,

    (A) DNA is directly responsible for the synthesis of a protein.

    (B) mRNA makes DNA.

    (C) transcription follows translation.

    (D) proteins are assemblages of amino acids.

33. Transcription can best be described as

    (A) the assembly of DNA from a protein model.

    (B) mRNA manufacture of a protein.

    (C) DNA manufacture of mRNA.

    (D) replication.

34. Relative to DNA, mRNA could be considered a

    (A) nucleotide.

    (B) duplicate of DNA.

    (C) replicate of DNA.

    (D) complement of DNA.

Passage for questions 35 to 40:

As far back as 1936, surgeons were working out a way to treat psychosis by an operation called prefrontal lobotomy—the last resort for schizophrenics and manic-depressives. Using a technique devised by the University of Lisbon's emeritus professor, Dr. Antonio Caetano de Abreu Freire Egas Moniz, skilled neurosurgeons cut away important nerve connections in the prefrontal brain lobe (a seat of reasoning) and the thalamus in the rear of the brain (a way station for emotional responses). The operation's aim: helping the patient to a better adjustment with his environment.

Working in a similar field was a 68-year-old Swiss physiologist, Dr. Walter Rudolph Hess, Director of Zurich University's Physiological Institute. A specialist in the circulatory and nervous systems, Dr. Hess studied the reaction of animals to electric shocks. By applying electrodes to parts of a cat's brain, he was able to make the animal do what it would normally do if it saw a dog, i.e., hiss, etc. By experimenting, Dr. Hess was able to determine how parts of the brain control organs of the body.

In 1949, the Council of the Caroline Institute at the University of Stockholm awarded the Nobel Prize in Medicine and Physiology jointly to Dr. Hess and Dr. Moniz. His half of the $30,000 would come in handy to Dr. Hess. Said he: "It will simplify my work. I have certain plans and everything costs money. . . . Now I will be able to hire assistants."

35. A prefrontal lobotomy is
    (A) a psychosis.
    (B) an operation on the brain.
    (C) a mental aberration.
    (D) a schizophrenic.

36. Prefrontal lobotomy is used on
    (A) skilled neurosurgeons.
    (B) mild cases of schizophrenia.
    (C) maladjusted people.
    (D) extreme cases of mental disease.

37. The prefrontal lobotomy involves
    (A) cutting the prefrontal brain lobe.
    (B) severing nerve connections.
    (C) destroying the thalamus.
    (D) massaging brain tissues.

38. As a result of a prefrontal lobotomy, doctors hope to
    (A) eliminate schizophrenia.
    (B) regenerate injured nerve tissue.
    (C) destroy germs which cause the disease.
    (D) help the patient get along better in normal life.

39. The operation is based on the theory that
    (A) people react to electric shock.
    (B) certain parts of the brain control certain types of action.
    (C) adjustment is a matter of proper reactions.
    (D) a dog will hiss if certain spots are touched with an electric wire.

40. Drs. Hess and Moniz jointly made news because
    (A) they did excellent work.
    (B) they effected wonderful cures.
    (C) they were awarded the Nobel Prize.
    (D) they effected a revolution in medical techniques.

Passage for questions 41 to 45:

Fluorine, chlorine, bromine, and iodine constitute an active group of nonmetals known as the *halogens*. Their degree of activity in combining with metals and hydrogen to form salts and acids respectively is represented by the order in which they were just given. Fluorine is the most active and iodine the least active in the series. They are found widely distributed in nature as salts. Examples of such salts are sodium chloride and calcium fluoride.

A *binary acid* is one that contains only two elements, hydrogen and a nonmetal. Halogens form binary acids, such as hydrochloric acid and hydrofluoric acid. The halogens can be prepared for laboratory study by the oxidation of their binary acids. Thus, when concentrated hydrochloric acid is oxidized by manganese dioxide, chlorine is given off.

All of the halogens contain seven electrons in their outer shell. In attempting to complete this outer shell, they act in such a way as to gain an electron. Elements (including oxygen) that attempt to gain electrons are called *oxidizing agents*. The halogens act as oxidizing agents in reaction with metals, hydrogen, and water.

The individual halogens can be identified as follows:

- Chlorine is a green-yellow gas which produces a light yellow color when mixed with carbon tetrachloride.

- Bromine is a red-brown liquid. When bromine is mixed with carbon tetrachloride, it produces an amber-colored solution.

- Iodine is a gray-colored solid. When mixed with carbon tetrachloride, it produces a violet-colored solution.

When a halogen is combined with another element, it is known as a *halide*. The halides can be identified as follows:

- When silver nitrate is added to chloride, a white precipitate is formed. This precipitate will dissolve in aluminum hydroxide but not in nitric acid.

- The test of a bromide is to dissolve the substance in water to which a small amount of chlorine water and carbon tetrachloride have been added. After the mixture is shaken and the layers have separated out, the carbon tetrachloride will settle to the bottom of the tube. If a bromide is present, the carbon tetrachloride layer will become orange in color.

- The procedure in testing for an iodide is the same as for a bromide. If an iodide is present, the carbon tetrachloride layer will become violet in color.

The halogens are of great importance in the modern world. Chlorine is used as a bleaching agent and a purifier of water. It is also used in antiseptic solutions, in gold extraction, and in the preparation of many organic compounds, such as DDT, chloroform, and synthetic rubber. Some of bromine's most important uses are in producing photographic paper, ethylene dibromide (used in making lead tetraethyl, the anti-knock ingredient in gasoline), and many kinds of drugs. Iodine is used in medicine, in the production of photographic film, and as an antiseptic. Fluorine's commercial uses include the etching of glass, the prevention of dental caries, and the production of refrigerants, plastics, insecticides, and lubricants.

The most useful of the halogen acids are hydrochloric and hydrofluoric acids. Hydrochloric acid has a great array of industrial uses, including the cleaning of metals (called *pickling*) and the manufacture of dyes and textiles. Hydrofluoric acid is widely used in the etching of glass and in the making of cryolite, a substance used in the extraction of aluminum from its ore.

41. A red-brown liquid is found in an unlabeled bottle. A few drops of carbon tetrachloride are added and the solution color turns amber. The liquid is

    (A) fluorine.

    (B) chlorine.

    (C) bromine.

    (D) iodine.

42. Binary acids are formed by

    (A) combining any two elements.

    (B) combining oxygen and a liquid.

    (C) combining hydrogen and a gas.

    (D) combining hydrogen and any nonmetal.

43. An oxidizing agent reacts with

    (A) metals, hydrogen, and water.

    (B) oxygen, halogen, and water.

    (C) electrons, metals, and elements.

    (D) carbon tetrachloride, nitric acid, and white precipitates.

44. Aluminum is extracted from its ore by

    (A) a process called pickling.

    (B) a substance named cryolite.

    (C) hydrochloric acid.

    (D) hydrofluoric acid.

45. An oxidizing agent behaves as it does in an attempt to

    (A) gain an eighth electron.

    (B) complete its inner core.

    (C) complete its outer shell.

    (D) get rid of as many electrons as possible.

End of Reading Comprehension Section

If you finish your work on this section before time is called, check your work on this section only. Do not return to any previous sections.

Sample Allied Health Professions Admission Test
Correct Answers

• •

VERBAL ABILITY

1. C	16. D	31. B	46. D	61. C
2. D	17. D	32. D	47. B	62. C
3. C	18. B	33. C	48. C	63. A
4. D	19. A	34. D	49. D	64. D
5. C	20. B	35. D	50. D	65. A
6. A	21. D	36. B	51. A	66. A
7. D	22. A	37. A	52. B	67. B
8. A	23. D	38. D	53. D	68. A
9. B	24. D	39. D	54. A	69. C
10. A	25. A	40. B	55. D	70. B
11. C	26. D	41. C	56. B	71. C
12. A	27. B	42. B	57. C	72. A
13. D	28. C	43. C	58. A	73. D
14. C	29. C	44. A	59. B	74. D
15. A	30. A	45. C	60. A	75. A

QUANTITATIVE ABILITY

1. D	8. D	15. A	22. A	29. B
2. D	9. D	16. D	23. B	30. D
3. D	10. B	17. D	24. C	31. C
4. B	11. C	18. C	25. D	32. D
5. D	12. D	19. A	26. B	33. D
6. A	13. D	20. D	27. D	34. C
7. B	14. A	21. C	28. D	35. D

36. D   39. A   42. C   45. A   48. C
37. C   40. C   43. B   46. C   49. D
38. D   41. B   44. A   47. C   50. B

BIOLOGY

1. C   11. D   21. D   31. D   41. B
2. C   12. D   22. B   32. D   42. D
3. A   13. C   23. C   33. B   43. B
4. D   14. B   24. B   34. B   44. D
5. B   15. D   25. D   35. B   45. D
6. B   16. A   26. A   36. A   46. A
7. D   17. C   27. C   37. A   47. C
8. A   18. D   28. A   38. A   48. B
9. C   19. D   29. B   39. A   49. B
10. C   20. A   30. D   40. C   50. C

CHEMISTRY

1. C   11. B   21. A   31. D   41. D
2. D   12. B   22. A   32. D   42. D
3. A   13. B   23. C   33. A   43. A
4. D   14. A   24. A   34. B   44. B
5. D   15. A   25. B   35. A   45. A
6. C   16. C   26. C   36. A   46. A
7. B   17. A   27. D   37. C   47. B
8. B   18. B   28. A   38. B   48. B
9. D   19. B   29. C   39. D   49. A
10. D   20. D   30. A   40. A   50. B

READING COMPREHENSION

1. D	10. A	19. C	28. B	37. B
2. A	11. C	20. A	29. B	38. D
3. D	12. B	21. D	30. C	39. B
4. D	13. D	22. C	31. A	40. C
5. B	14. A	23. C	32. D	41. C
6. A	15. D	24. B	33. C	42. D
7. B	16. D	25. A	34. D	43. A
8. C	17. A	26. D	35. B	44. B
9. B	18. C	27. C	36. D	45. C

Explanatory Answers

. . . .

VERBAL ABILITY

1. **(C)** One who is *delinquent* neglects to do what is required or, at least, fails to do it on time. The best synonym offered for *delinquent* is *late*. A juvenile delinquent is a youthful person who does not meet expectations. Juvenile delinquents may be lawless and violent, but the word *delinquent* refers to their failure to do what duty or law requires.
   Example: If you are delinquent in paying your taxes, you must pay a fine.

2. **(D)** To *proscribe* is to forbid by law. The impact of the word is much stronger than to merely deny. The word meaning *explain* is *describe*. That which is proscribed may be published, but the proscription is the prohibition itself.
   Example: Employment of undocumented aliens is proscribed by federal legislation.

3. **(C)** *Clemency* is *leniency* or *mercy*. Clemency should not be confused with *amnesty*, which is *pardon*. With respect to the sentencing of convicted defendants, clemency entails a lighter sentence whereas amnesty implies immediate release.
   Example: In light of his client's family responsibilities, the attorney requested clemency of the judge.

4. **(D)** To *rehabilitate* is to restore a former state or capacity. Rehabilitation may involve all three other choices to a greater or lesser extent, but the purpose of the training, replacement, and/or compensation is to restore to previous function.
   Example: The goal of physical therapy is rehabilitation of the injured limb.

5. **(C)** *Cursory* means *hurried* or *superficial*. It has nothing to do with profanity, verbal abuse, or cursing. The word that refers to flowing handwriting is *cursive*.

Example: In a cursory search of the premises, the police officer found no sign of the murder weapon.

6. **(A)** *Tacit* means not expressed openly but implied or silently agreed to. The other choices all have very different meanings. *Concisely* means *tersely*; *delicately* is a definition of *tactfully*; and *tangibly* refers to the *tactile* sense.
   Example: Nothing was written in the bylaws, but by tacit agreement of the members of the board, no minority applicants were admitted to the club.

7. **(D)** *Indigent* means *poor, needy*, or *destitute*. The commonly used term "indigent poor" is a redundancy. The word meaning *angry* is *indignant*. The word meaning *lazy* is *indolent*.
   Example: In times of high inflation, the indigent suffer both hunger and homelessness.

8. **(A)** *Stringent* means *strict, severe*, or *rigid*. Stringency does not necessarily imply harshness or unfairness. The word meaning *cleansing* is *astringent*.
   Example: Betting on sporting events is governed by stringent rules.

9. **(B)** *Pecuniary* refers to *financial* or *monetary* matters. As to the other choices: *strange* is *peculiar*; *special* is *particular*; and *intense* is *purposeful*.
   Example: The mediator should be a disinterested party with no pecuniary interest in the outcome of the negotiations.

10. **(A)** To *tabulate* is to *arrange* data in a *systematic manner*. All the other choices may enter into the tabulation of the data, but they do not serve as synonyms; they are not the same thing.
    Example: The election data were tabulated by

township and entered in neat columns on a master chart.

11. **(C)** A *facsimile* is an *exact copy*. A *forgery* is meant to substitute for the real thing rather than to serve as a copy. Anything less than an exact copy is not a facsimile.
Example: The photocopying machine produces many facsimiles with great speed.

12. **(A)** To *peruse* is to *read carefully*, to *scrutinize*, or to *study*. To *seize* is to *preempt*; to *stroll* is to *perambulate*; to *spindle* is to *perforate*.
Example: Peruse every clause in the contract before you sign it.

13. **(D)** *Larceny* is the legal term for *theft*. Burglary, robbery, and embezzlement are all forms of larceny.
Example: The perpetrators of the stock fraud were charged with grand larceny.

14. **(C)** *Noxious* means *harmful*, *injurious*, or *unwholesome*. The adjective *noxious* often appears with the noun "fumes" or "odor." Noxious fumes may smell unpleasant, but what makes them noxious is the harmful aspect.
Example: The noxious fumes from the refinery poisoned the air.

15. **(A)** To *apprise* is to *inform* or to *give notice to*. Apprisal often involves giving warning, but not necessarily. The word meaning to *judge* is *appraise*; that meaning *repeat* is *reprise*.
Example: When police officers take a suspect into custody, they must apprise the suspect of his or her right to remain silent.

16. **(D)** The word *fiscal* means relating to financial matters in general. *Inherited* could be viewed as slightly related since inheritance often involves financial matters. However, the basic meaning of *inherited*—received by inheritance—is completely different from the meaning of *fiscal*.
Example: Fiscal problems caused the hospital to abandon its play therapy program.

17. **(D)** *Interim* refers to something that is effective for an interval of time. *Temporary* refers to something that lasts for only a limited time. *Permanent* is opposite in meaning.
Example: The acting director will serve on an interim basis until a permanent replacement can be found.

18. **(B)** To *collaborate* is to work with another, especially on a project of mutual interest. *Work independently* is opposite in meaning.
Example: Allied health professionals often collaborate in their service to clients.

19. **(A)** To be *altruistic* means to be concerned for or devoted to the welfare of others. *Extended* could be viewed as slightly related, since *altruistic* people often extend themselves to help others. However, the basic meaning of *extended*—stretched out—is completely different from the meaning of *altruistic*. A vague connection exists between *altruistic* and *appealing*. *Altruistic* people often make appeals on behalf of those less fortunate than themselves. Simultaneously, the generosity of *altruistic* people often makes them very *appealing* to other people. Although this vague connection exists between *altruistic* and *appealing*, they do not share a similar meaning.
Example: The altruistic podiatrist volunteers one afternoon each week at the neighborhood senior citizens' center.

20. **(B)** The word *fraudulent* means characterized by deceit or trickery, especially deliberate misrepresentation. *Suspicious*—sensing that something is wrong without definite proof—could describe a person's reaction to a *fraudulent* situation. *Unfair* and *despicable*, could both be used to describe a *fraudulent* act. However, the basic meanings of these words are completely different from the meaning of *fraudulent*.
Example: An unscrupulous person may obtain controlled substances through use of fraudulent prescriptions.

21. **(D)** An *allegation* is a declaration that something is true, sometimes with little or no proof. An *asser-*

tion is an affirmation that something is true. *Denial* is opposite in meaning to *allegation*. A *denial* is a declaration that something is false.

Example: The prisoner made the allegation that he had been beaten in the station house.

22. **(A)** The word *stipulation* refers to a required condition or item specified in a contract, treaty, or other official document. A *stipulation* could be an *addition* to a contract or other document, but even without *unnecessary*, response B is incorrect. *Required correction* shares with *stipulation* the idea of being necessary as well as an association with something written. However, a *correction* is an alteration made to remedy or remove an error or fault, so its basic meaning is completely different from that of *stipulation*.

Example: The scholarship was granted with the stipulation that the dental hygienist work for two years in an underserved area.

23. **(D)** *Allocation* is the act of setting something apart for a particular purpose. To *site* means to put something in a location or position; however, the emphasis with *site* is on the physical location given to an object rather than on the purpose of the object.

Example: In difficult economic times, many agencies compete for allocation of funds for their own projects.

24. **(D)** The word *perennial* means lasting through a succession of years or through a long, indefinite, or infinite time. Therefore, *enduring* is the best synonym. *Changeable* is opposite in meaning to *perennial*. Responses B and C share the general idea of time with *perennial*, but the specific meanings of *frequent* and *occasional* are completely different from that of *perennial*.

Example: Ticks and fleas are a perennial problem for dogs that spend much time out of doors, especially in summer.

25. **(A)** *Emissions* refers to anything sent or given forth from a source, including gases, liquids, solids, and energy. *Embassies* shares the idea of sending forth, but it refers to people entrusted with accomplishing a mission. *Approaches* is almost opposite in mean-

ing to *emissions*. *Trends* is only slightly related in that it involves general movement, but its basic meaning is completely different from that of *emissions*.

Example: Automobile emissions controls have been very effective in cutting down urban air pollution.

26. **(D)** The word *rhetorical* means characterized by artificial eloquence, especially by a showy or elaborate style. Therefore, *grandiloquent* is the best synonym. *Inquisitive* is unrelated to the meaning of *rhetorical* except perhaps by association with the phrase "a *rhetorical* question." Responses B and C share the idea of speech with *rhetorical* however, both *laconic* and *tacit* have opposite meanings, respectively, "brief or terse in speech" and "implicitly stated."

Example: The orator asked many rhetorical questions strictly for effect; he did not expect any answers.

27. **(B)** *Rudimentary* refers to the fundamental elements or first principles of a subject. Response A, *classic*, shares the idea of firstness with *rudimentary* in that one of the meanings of *classic* is being of the first or highest quality. However, the two words are almost opposite in meaning and usage.

Example: The new lab assistant had a rudimentary knowledge of the requirements of the job but needed lots of experience and training in order to gain full understanding.

28. **(C)** *Salutary* means *beneficial*, *remedial*, or *curative*. The word which means *welcoming* is *salutatory*. The choice of *forceful* might stem from your associating with *salute*, but *salute* and *salutary* are in no way related.

Example: After a long bout with the flu, a trip to a warm climate might have a salutary effect upon your health.

29. **(C)** To *acquiesce* is to *agree quietly* or to *consent*. If you chose *inquire*, you probably saw *question* in *quiesc*. Reading carefully is an important component of answering vocabulary questions.

Example: A therapist must sometimes acquiesce

to the procedures outlined by the doctor in order to present a united front to the patient.

30. (A) *Diffidence* is *lack of self-confidence* or *shyness*. The word is in no way related to *indifference*, which is *unconcern*, nor to *difference*.
Example: The diffident child was able to express herself best at the painting easel.

31. (B) To *capitulate* is to *stop resisting* or to *surrender*. *Retreat* may well be a component of *capitulation*, but not necessarily. Avoid confusion with *recap*, which would mean *repeat*, or with *capitalization*, which would refer to *financing*.
Example: With patience you might be able to convince the elderly gentleman to capitulate and to take his medicine.

32. (D) *Auspicious* means *attended by good omens* or *favorable*. It has nothing to do with *suspicious* or *questionable*.
Example: The accident victim's quick return to consciousness was an auspicious sign for a total recovery.

33. (C) *Access* is *entrance* or *admittance*. It is NOT the same as *excess*.
Example: Only authorized personnel are permitted access to the storage room.

34. (D) That which is *cogent* is *well-reasoned, valid*, and *convincing*. It is the opposite of *confused* or *unintentional*.
Example: The veterinarian presented a number of cogent arguments for putting the sick dog to sleep.

35. (D) *Ostensibly* means *apparently*. Use of this word does leave some room for doubt.
Example: Ostensibly it is easier to adjust to graduated lenses than to bifocals.

36. (B) *Answer*. A *query* is a question.

37. (A) *Benevolent* means full of generous and kind feelings. *Vitriolic* means caustic and bitter in feeling or speech.

38. (D) *Open-minded. Myopic* means narrow-minded or shortsighted. "Myopia" is nearsightedness.

39. (D) *Smooth. Napped* means having a hairy or downy surface, as suede.

40. (B) *Antagonize* means to provoke hostility. *Placate* means to soothe or mollify.

41. (C) *Talkative. Reticent* means uncommunicative in speech.

42. (B) *Exclusive* means limiting or restricting. *Eclectic* means accepting from many different sources.

43. (C) *Perpetuate* means to cause to last indefinitely. *Expunge* means to destroy.

44. (A) *Supine* means lying flat on the back. *Ambulatory* means walking about.

45. (C) *Expedite* means to execute promptly. *Procrastinate* means to put off intentionally.

46. (D) *Paranoid* means suspicious. *Intrepid* means fearless.

47. (B) *Result*. The *result* is the end product of a *cause*. A synonym for *result* is *effect*. Do not confuse *effect* with *affect*, which means influence.

48. (C) That which is *inane* is empty and pointless. That which is *pithy* has substance and point.

49. (D) *Urban* means pertaining to a city or town. *Rural* pertains to the country, especially agricultural areas. *Suburban* and *exurban* fall between the opposites.

50. (D) *Death. Birth* is the beginning of a continuum that ends in *death*.

51. (A) *Bestial* means as brutal as an animal. *Humane* means kind and benevolent.

52. **(B)** *Soft*. *Weak* might also be considered an antonym for *hard*, but it is not as clear and definite an antonym as *soft*. You must choose the *best* answer.

53. **(D)** *Alkaline* is the chemical opposite of *acid*. *Alkalis* neutralize *acids*.

54. **(A)** *Patient*. *Brusque* means abrupt and short in manner.

55. **(D)** *Concrete* means specific or particular. *Abstract* means general or theoretical.

56. **(B)** *Gluttony* means excessive eating. *Anorexia* means self-starvation.

57. **(C)** *Floor*. The *roof* and *foundation* are opposites, being the extreme outer limits of a building. The *floor* and *ceiling* are opposites within a room.

58. **(A)** *Fusion* means blending together. *Fission* means breaking into parts. The two processes, while total opposites, can both create nuclear energy.

59. **(B)** *Bend*. To *freeze* is to stiffen. The antonym you choose must be the same part of speech as the original word. The antonym of the verb to *freeze*, meaning to chill, would be to *heat*. "Hot" is the opposite of "cold," not of "freeze."

60. **(A)** *Urbane*. *Provincial* means unsophisticated.

61. **(C)** *Clerical* means related to the clergy or to the church. *Secular* means civil and in no way connected to a church.

62. **(C)** *Lethargy* is inaction or indifference. *Verve* is great vitality.

63. **(A)** *Slick*. *Glutinous* means sticky or gummy.

64. **(D)** *Mound*. A *grotto* is a cave.

65. **(A)** *Barren*. *Verdant* means green and lush with vegetation.

66. **(A)** *Fearlessness*. *Trepidation* means fear.

67. **(B)** *Reinstate*. To *rescind* is to take back, so the *best* antonym is a reversal of the process. *Provide* might serve as an antonym if there were no better choice.

68. **(A)** *Addition*. *Abatement* means diminution.

69. **(C)** *Aloof*. One who is *officious* is meddlesome and bossy. One who is *aloof* takes no interest in the affairs of others.

70. **(B)** *Hawk*. Birds cannot be opposites of one another, nor can one really say that a bird is the opposite of an animal. To answer this antonym question, you must think of the birds as symbols. The *dove* is a symbol of peace; its opposite is the *hawk*, a symbol of war.

71. **(C)** *Pure*. *Adulterated* means corrupt.

72. **(A)** *Fatigue*. *Stamina* is endurance.

73. **(D)** *Rigid*. *Supple* means flexible.

74. **(D)** *Repression*. *Catharsis* is emotional release.

75. **(A)** *Impartiality*. *Nepotism* is favoritism shown to relatives.

QUANTITATIVE ABILITY

1. (D) Since the quotient, when multiplied by 617, must give 333,180 as an answer, the quotient must end in a number which, when multiplied by 617, will end in 0. This can only be (D), since 617 times (A) would end in 7, (B) would end in 4, and (C) in 3.

2. (D) The sum of the digits in both the numerator and denominator are divisible by 9.

3. (D) $3^\circ + 9^{1/2} + (1/3)^{-2} = 1 + 3 + 9 = 13$

4. (B) $\dfrac{(+4) + 0 + (-1) + (-5) + (-8)}{5} = \dfrac{-10}{5} = -2$

5. (D) Compare $2\pi r$ with $2\pi(r + 3)$.
$2\pi(r + 3) = 2\pi r + 6\pi$
Circumference was increased by 6π. Trying this with a numerical value for r will give the same result.

6. (A) In the table, the angle whose cosine is closest to .4000 is 66°.

7. (B) $\dfrac{9}{11} - \dfrac{3}{5} = \dfrac{45 - 33}{55} = \dfrac{12}{55}$

8. (D) $\dfrac{6x + 5y - (4x + y)}{2x} = \dfrac{6x + 5y - 4x - y}{2x} =$

$\dfrac{2x + 4y}{2x} = \dfrac{2(x + 2y)}{2x} = \dfrac{x + 2y}{x}$

9. (D) $4\sqrt{27} = 4\sqrt{9}\sqrt{3} = 12\sqrt{3}$
$2\sqrt{48} = 2\sqrt{16}\sqrt{3} = 8\sqrt{3}$
$\sqrt{147} = \sqrt{49}\sqrt{3} = 7\sqrt{3}$
$12\sqrt{3} - 8\sqrt{3} + 7\sqrt{3} = 11\sqrt{3}$

10. (B) Area of parallelogram = b • h
$(x + 7)(x - 7) = 15$
$x^2 - 49 = 15$
$x^2 = 64$
$x = 8$
Base = x + 7 = 15

11. (C) $\cos 68^\circ = \dfrac{NP}{4}$
$NP = 4 \cos 68^\circ$
$NP = 4(.3746) = 1.5$ to the nearest tenth

12. (D) $\dfrac{7}{8} \cdot \dfrac{2}{3} \cdot \dfrac{8}{1} = \dfrac{14}{3}$

13. (D) $(2x - 3)(3x + 5) = 6x^2 + 10x - 9x - 15$
$= 6x^2 + x - 15$

14. (A) $\begin{array}{r} 61 \quad = 60^{12}/_{12} \\ -45^5/_{12} = 45^5/_{12} \\ \hline 15^7/_{12} \end{array}$

15. (A) $2\sqrt{18} \cdot 6\sqrt{2} = 12\sqrt{36} = 12 \cdot 6 = 72$

16. (D) Arrange the grades in order:
0, 1, 4, 4, 4, 5, 5, 5, 7, 7, 7, 7, 8, 9, 9, 10, 10
There are 17 grades. The ninth (middle) grade is 7.

17. (D) The grade of 7 appears four times, more than any other grade.

18. (C) $V = \pi r^2 h = {}^{22}/_7 \cdot 49 \cdot 10 = 1540$ cubic inches
Divide by 231 to find gallons.

19. (A)

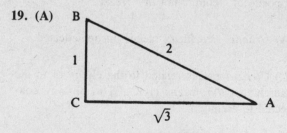

If $\sin A = 1/2$, $\sin B = \dfrac{\sqrt{3}}{2}$

20. (D) Use a common denominator of 60.
${}^5/_{12} = {}^{25}/_{60}$; ${}^8/_{15} = {}^{32}/_{60}$
${}^7/_{15} = {}^{28}/_{60}$; ${}^{31}/_{60}$
Since $1/2 = {}^{30}/_{60}$, the answer closest to $1/2$ is (D).

21. (C)

$\angle 1 + \angle 3 = 180°$
$\angle 3 + \angle 2$
Therefore, $\angle 1 + \angle 2 = 180°$

22. (A) $2(a - b) + 4(a + 3b) = 2a - 2b + 4a + 12b$
$= 6a + 10b$

23. (B) $\dfrac{3x^2(x - y)}{9x(x - y)} = \dfrac{x}{3}$

24. (C) $\dfrac{5}{12} \cdot 100 = \dfrac{125}{3} = 41\dfrac{2}{3}\%$
To change a fraction to a percent, multiply by 100.

25. (D) Represent the angles as x, 5x, and 6x. They must add to 180°.
$12x = 180$
$x = 15$
The angles are 15°, 75°, and 90°.

26. (B) 24 minutes is $^{24}/_{60}$ or $^2/_5$ of an hour.

27. (D) The integers are 3, 13, 23, 33, 43. Since these are evenly spaced, the average is the middle integer, 23.

28. (D) An angle outside the circle is $^1/_2$ the difference of its intercepted arcs.

29. (B)

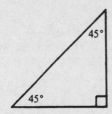

$\sec 45° = \dfrac{1}{\cos 45°}$

$= \dfrac{1}{\frac{\sqrt{2}}{2}} = \dfrac{2}{\sqrt{2}} \cdot \dfrac{\sqrt{2}}{\sqrt{2}} = \dfrac{2\sqrt{2}}{2} = \sqrt{2}$

30. (D) $(a - b)^2 = a^2 - 2ab + b^2 = 40$
Substituting 8 for ab, we have
$a^2 - 16 + b^2 = 40$
$a^2 + b^2 = 56$

31. (C) $^1/_5\% = .2\% = .002$
$40 \cdot .002 = .0800$

32. (D) $\tan B = \dfrac{\text{opposite}}{\text{adjacent}}$
By the Pythagorean Theorem, the length of the side adjacent to $\angle B$ is given by

$x^2 + (6\sqrt{3})^2 = 12^2$
$x^2 + 108 = 144$
$x^2 = 36$
$x = 6$

Thus, $\tan B = \dfrac{6\sqrt{3}}{6} = \sqrt{3}$

33. (D) $12\frac{1}{2}\% = ^1/_8 \quad ^1/_8 \cdot 160 = \$20$ discount
New sale price = \$140
$3\% = ^3/_{100} \quad ^3/_{100} \cdot 140 = ^{420}/_{100} = \$4.20$
second discount
\$135.80 final sale price
Therefore \$160 - \$135.80 or \$24.20 was saved.

34. (C) Since the last digit is 9, the square root must end in 3 or 7.

35. (D) 86° is 2 above the average of 84
82° is 2 below
90° is 6 above
92° is 8 above
80° is 4 below
81° is 3 below
So far, there are 16° above and 9° below. Therefore the missing term is 7° below the average, or 77°.

36. (D) $80 = ^1/_8 x$
$640 = x$

37. (C)

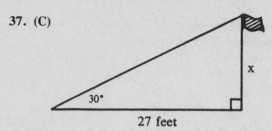

$$\tan 30° = \frac{x}{27}$$

$$\frac{\sqrt{3}}{3} = \frac{x}{27} \text{(cross-multiply)}$$

$$3x = 27\sqrt{3}$$

$$x = 9\sqrt{3} \text{ feet}$$

38. (D) $8 - 4a + 4 = 2 + 12 - 3a$
$12 - 4a = 14 - 3a$
$-2 = a$

39. (A)

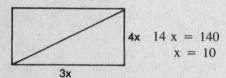

$14 x = 140$
$x = 10$

The rectangle is 30′ by 40′. This is a 3, 4, 5 right triangle, so the diagonal is 50′.

40. (C) $^4/_{80} = {}^1/_{20} \cdot 100 = 5\%$

41. (B) Multiply first equation by 3, second by 2, then subtract.
$$\begin{aligned} 6x + 9y &= 36b \\ \underline{6x - 2y} &= \underline{14b} \\ 11y &= 22b \\ y &= 2b \end{aligned}$$

42. (C) A hexagon has 6 sides.
Sum $= (n - 2)\,180 = 4(180) = 720$

43. (B) $(x - 10)(x + 2) = 0$
$x - 10 = 0 \quad x + 2 = 0$
$x = 10 \text{ or } -2$

44. (A) $36 = 1\frac{1}{2}x$
$36 = {}^3/_2x$
$72 = 3x$
$x = 24$

45. (A) Let x = number of dimes
$4x$ = number of quarters
$10x$ = value of dimes in cents
$100x$ = value of quarters in cents
$$\begin{aligned} 10x + 100x &= 220 \\ 110x &= 220 \\ x &= 2 \end{aligned}$$

46. (C)

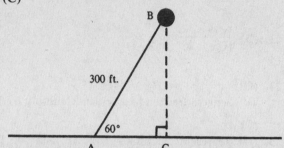

The distance from the balloon to the ground is indicated by the line segment BC in the drawing above.

Since $\sin A = \dfrac{\text{opposite}}{\text{hypotenuse}} = \dfrac{BC}{300}$

$$\sin 60° = \frac{BC}{300}$$

$$BC = 300\,(\sin 60°) = 300\left(\frac{\sqrt{3}}{2}\right) = 150\sqrt{3}$$

47. (C) Let x = Stephen's age now
$4x$ = Mark's age now
$x + 1$ = Stephen's age in 1 year
$4x + 1$ = Mark's age in 1 year

$4x + 1 = 3(x + 1)$
$4x + 1 = 3x + 3$
$x = 2$

Mark is now 8, so 2 years ago he was 6.

48. (C) $3(60) = 180$
$4(55) = 220$
$$7\overline{)400}$$
$57^1/_7$ which is 57.1 to the nearest tenth.

49. (D) If the dimensions are all doubled, the area is multiplied by 2^2 or 4. If the new area is 4 times as great as the original area, it has been *increased* by 300%.

50. **(B)**

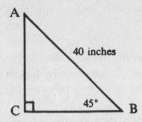

If the ball rolls from point A to point B, which is 40 inches, the distance the ball travels vertically is given by AC.

To determine AC:

$$\sin B = \frac{\text{opposite}}{\text{hypotenuse}} = \frac{AC}{40}$$

$$\sin 45° = \frac{AC}{40}$$

$$40 \sin 45° = AC$$

$$40 \left(\frac{\sqrt{2}}{2}\right) = AC$$

Thus, $AC = 20\sqrt{2}$

BIOLOGY

1. **(C)** Offspring that contain the n allele would be all heterozygotes (Nn) and homozygote recessives (nn). Homozygote dominants (NN) would comprise $.8 \times .8 = .64$, and thus the remainder (.36) would contain n. Alternatively, we could calculate the number of homozygote recessives ($.2 \times .2 = .04$) and add them to the number of heterozygotes ($.2 \times .8 \times 2 = .32$) and derive .36.

2. **(C)** All chordates possess a notochord at some point during their life span.

3. **(A)** Most bryophytes have no vascular tissue. They do require water for fertilization and have a dominant multicellular haploid stage.

4. **(D)** Skeletal, striated, and voluntary are all names for the same kind of muscle, that which produces movement of most external appendages. Smooth muscle comprises the walls of internal organs.

5. **(B)** Saprophytes live and feed on dead organic matter. Mushrooms are saprophytes.

6. **(B)** Its great length, numerous folds, and absorptive villi and microvilli are some of the structural adaptations of the small intestine for digestive absorption.

7. **(D)** Ribosomes are the organelles where polypeptide chains are formed from amino acids.

8. **(A)** Only viruses may have genes composed of double-stranded DNA, single-stranded DNA, double-stranded RNA, or single-stranded RNA.

9. **(C)** Use of ATP is one characteristic that distinguishes bacteria from viruses. Some bacteria are photosynthetic, most reproduce through binary fission, and no bacteria have mitochondria.

10. **(C)** White blood cells, or leukocytes, remove foreign substances from the body. An infection would be revealed by a higher white blood cell count.

11. **(D)** The retina contains the receptor cells: the light-sensitive rods and the color-sensitive cones.

12. **(D)** Mitosis is the process by which the nucleus divides to produce two daughter nuclei, each with the same number of chromosomes as the diploid parent cell.

13. **(C)** Crossing over occurs during zygote formation in the first prophase of meiosis. At this time, genetic material is exchanged between homologous chromosomes of the mother and father.

14. **(B)** Since the glucose would be going against the concentration gradient, a net expenditure of energy would be required; this is active transport. Passive transport and osmosis require no expenditure of energy.

15. **(D)** A person who does not have Down's syndrome has 23 pairs of chromosomes, or 46 chromosomes. Down's syndrome results from non-disjunction of chromosome 21. Because an additional chromosome is inherited, each somatic cell will contain 47 chromosomes.

16. **(A)** For the daughter to express a recessive sex-linked trait, she must receive a copy of the recessive allele from both parents. Since the mother does not possess the recessive allele, the daughter cannot be color-blind. A son, on the other hand, would have a 50% chance of being color-blind; if he inherited the copy of this allele from his father, he would be color-blind, and if he inherited it from his mother he would not be.

17. **(C)** Deoxygenated blood will flow from the anterior and posterior vena cavae into the right ventricle of the heart and follow the sequence indicated in choice (C). It picks up oxygen in pulmonary capillaries (between the pulmonary veins and pulmonary artery) and pumps oxygenated blood back out to the body from the aorta.

18. **(D)** Glucose is the end product of photosynthesis. ADP is needed to synthesize the ATP needed to power photosynthetic reactions. Chlorophyll traps the solar energy needed to split water. Oxygen released during the reaction comes from carbon dioxide.

19. **(D)** RNA has uracil rather than thymine as one of its pyrimidine bases. Uracil will bond with adenine during DNA transcription.

20. **(A)** Transfer RNA carries amino acids to the ribosomes during protein synthesis. mRNA is transcribed in the nucleus and carries information to the ribosomes that dictates which proteins will be synthesized. Most of the length of mRNA is introns, regions that do not code for specific amino acids.

21. **(D)** During aerobic respiration, oxygen serves as the final acceptor for hydrogen released from glucose and other organic molecules.

22. **(B)** When parents bearing two different homozygous characters are crossed and only one phenotype of the character results, that character must be dominant in the heterozygote form. Here, SS × ss ◗ Ss offspring, but S (Smooth) must be dominant over s (wrinkled).

23. **(C)** The nerve cell membrane must be polarized so that sodium can rush into the cell and potassium can rush out during transmission of a nerve impulse. Choices A and B dampen propagation of a nerve impulse.

24. **(B)** Geographic isolation is thought to be a requirement for most speciation events. Sympatric populations are not geographically separated. Thus sympatry is an impediment to speciation.

25. **(D)** Only mammals have three bones in the middle ear: the malleus, incus, and stapes. Some other vertebrates (for example, some fish) bear live young, and some mammals (monotremes) lay eggs. Birds are endothermic and have four-chambered hearts.

26. **(A)** The archenteron will later become the cavity of the digestive tract. It forms during gastrulation and is below the neural groove.

27. **(C)** Enzymes are proteins that act as catalysts for reactions in biological systems.

28. **(A)** A hypertonic medium is one that has a higher concentration than the cell. A cell in a hypertonic medium will lose water by osmosis to the hypertonic medium and will shrink.

29. **(B)** The T cells are produced in the thymus and are lymphocytes that respond to large foreign antigens such as cancer cells and virus-infected cells.

30. **(D)** The sporophyte is the diploid phase of the organism, and is the dominant phase in land plants. Pollen and protective seeds are adaptations against dessication in the land environment.

31. **(D)** The ovary contains the seed, which is an embryo contained in a ripened ovule.

32. **(D)** Cell division leaves ribosomes unchanged. Centrioles, nuclei, and mitochondria are radically changed during mitosis.

33. **(B)** These are the distinguishing characteristics of crustaceans.

34. **(B)** The cell vacuole is a storage compartment and contains no DNA.

35. **(B)** Cleavage is the process of repeated mitotic cell divisions by which the fertilized egg develops into a multicellular embryo.

36. **(A)** FSH, follicle stimulating hormone, stimulates the follicles in the ovary to produce eggs. FSH is produced in the pituitary gland.

37. **(A)** In independent assortment, two traits are inherited independently. Hair color and eye color in this question are inherited independently.

38. **(A)** mRNA is transcribed from nuclear DNA, then moves out of the nucleus to the ribosomes, which bind to the endoplasmic reticulum. Newly synthesized enzymes move to the golgi apparatus, where they are repackaged into vesicles called lysosomes. Lysosomes excrete the enzymes into the cytosol.

39. **(A)** All seeds in the F_1 generation will have the genotype R/rG/g. Since wrinkled and green are the dominant traits, they will mask the recessive traits in the heterozygote form, and all offspring will appear wrinkled and green.

40. **(C)** When we cross RrGg × RrGg, we get 9R/-G/- (wrinkled green) : 3r/rG/- (wrinkled yellow) : 3R/-g/g (smooth green) : 1 r/r g/g (smooth yellow). The dash means that the second allele may be ei-

ther the dominant or the recessive one. Since at least one copy of the dominant allele is present, these progeny will bear the phenotype of the dominant allele.

41. **(B)** The limbic system is a group of areas of the brain that control emotion and feeling.

42. **(D)** The ulna is a bone in the forearm.

43. **(B)** The Hardy-Weinberg law says that under stable conditions, allelic frequencies will not change in successive generations of sexually reproducing organisms. In natural environments, these conditions are seldom met. Choice B is the opposite of Hardy-Weinberg requirements: mating must be completely random with respect to genotype.

44. **(D)** With environmental change comes natural selection for traits that are adaptive to the new environmental conditions.

45. **(D)** Equation D is the net result of aerobic respiration, a process that results in 38 ATP molecules being formed. Equations B and C are photosynthetic reactions. Equation A is anaerobic respiration, which results in the production of 2 ATP molecules.

46. **(A)** The gall bladder stores bile produced by the liver. Bile is used to emulsify fats.

47. **(C)** Homologous structures have common evolutionary and embryological origins. Analogous structures may not have common evolutionary or embryological origins but may only serve similar functions.

48. **(B)** Organelles adapted for storage of water, food, and toxic waste are called vacuoles.

49. **(B)** Potato starch and glycogen are both polysaccharides composed of many bonded glucose molecules.

50. **(C)** 50% of human offspring are boys and 50% are girls. How many girls or boys are already in the family is irrelevant.

CHEMISTRY

1. **(C)** The atomic mass or mass number of an atom is the sum of the number of neutrons and the number of protons in a nucleus.

2. **(D)** The first three statements summarize John Dalton's account of the laws of chemical change. Statement D was the conclusion of Rutherford's experiments many years later.

3. **(A)** Sulfur's atomic number of 16 indicates that it has 16 electrons distributed as $1s^2 2s^2 2p^6 3s^2 3p^4$. Thus sulfur has six 2p electrons.

4. **(D)** Electrons in higher sublevels than those they normally occupy are said to be in an excited state. In choice D, a 2p electron was "promoted" to a 3s electron.

5. **(D)** Elements with an atomic number greater than 83 have no known stable isotopes.

6. **(C)** When electrons fall back to a lower energy level, excess energy is released. The correct choice must indicate a drop in energy level, from the p-sublevel to the s-sublevel, or from the f-sublevel to the d-sublevel. In choice C, electrons are falling from the 3p to the 3s sublevel.

7. **(B)** The formula $A_x B_y$ represents a compound where there are x atoms of A for every y atoms of B. The compound represented by the formula $C_6H_{12}O_6$ has 12 atoms of hydrogen for every six atoms of carbon, for a ratio of 2 atoms of hydrogen to 1 atom of carbon.

8. **(B)** Because of the relationship between moles and atoms, the molecular formula of a compound provides information about the relative number of moles of atoms in the compound. In $A_x B_y$, there are x moles of A for every y moles of B. The compound represented by the formula $C_6H_{12}O_6$ has 12 moles of hydrogen for every 6 moles of carbon, for a ratio of 2 moles of hydrogen to 1 mole of carbon.

9. **(D)** Gram molecular mass equals the sum of gram atomic masses of the atoms in the formula. Remember that the gram atomic mass is approximately double the element's number on the periodic table because of the mass of protons and neutrons in each atom. Here, C = 12 and O = (2 × 16) = 32, or 44 grams/mole. The question specifies 4 moles, or 4 × 44 = 176.

10. **(D)** One mole of any ideal gas occupies 22.4 liters at standard temperature and pressure (STP). According to Boyle's Law, when temperature remains constant, the volume of a gas is inversely related to the amount of pressure applied on it. When the pressure is halved, the volume doubles: 2 × 22.4 = 44.8.

11. **(B)** A balanced chemical equation has the same numbers and kinds of atoms on each side of the equation. The 2 oxygen atoms to the left of the arrow must be balanced by a coefficient of 2 for water on the right side of the arrow ($2H_2O$). A coefficient of 2 must then be added to hydrogen ($2H_2$) on the left. The balanced formula would be $2H_2 + Fe_3O_2 \rightarrow 3Fe + 2H_2O$.

12. **(B)** Sodium (Na) has atomic number 11 and atomic mass 22. Chlorine (Cl) has atomic number 17 and atomic mass 34. The total atomic mass of NaCl is 22 + 34 = 56. Sodium makes up 22/56 × 100, or just under 40% of the mass of NaCl.

13. **(B)** Avogadro's number, $6 × 10^{23}$, is the number of molecules in one mole of any substance.

14. **(A)** Ionic bonds are favored between elements at the left of the periodic table, like Mg, that have low ionization potentials and elements at the right of the periodic table, like Cl, that have high electron affinity.

15. **(A)** Energy is always released when bonds are formed.

16. **(C)** Chlorine has 7 valence electrons in its outer shell and when two atoms come together, a covalent bond will form where electrons are shared. Energy is always released when bonds form, and van der Waals forces are present in all matter.

17. **(A)** Hydrogen bonds form between H and F, Cl, Br, and I in descending order of strength. Thus HF has the strongest bonds of the four choices.

18. **(B)** An element's electronegativity is its tendency to attract shared electrons. In general, electronegativity decreases from left to right of the periodic table.

19. **(B)** Metals comprise more than 2/3 of the elements in the periodic table.

20. **(D)** At room temperature, only mercury (Hg) and bromine (Br) are liquids.

21. **(A)** The most active metal will most readily lose its valence electrons. The most active metals are found in Group IA, in the first column of the period table. Na is a group IA metal.

22. **(A)** Chlorine is a halogen (Group VII on the periodic table). Halogens are nonmetals and thus are poor conductors of electricity and heat. They tend to form acidic compounds.

23. **(C)** To solve this problem, use the formula: Calories = g H_2O × Change in Temperature × Specific Heat of H_2O. Substituting values, Calories = 100 × 5 × 1 = 500 calories.

24. **(A)** In an endothermic phase change, energy is absorbed. Liquid must be heated before it will change into a gas, and this process requires absorption of energy.

25. **(B)** When a liquid vaporizes, it becomes a gas. At vaporization point, temperature (and average kinetic energy) remain constant. The heat being gained represents a gain in potential energy. Gases have more potential energy than liquids, so when a liquid vaporizes, a gain in potential energy results.

26. **(C)** According to Boyle's Law, volume of a gas is inversely proportional to pressure exerted on the gas. Standard pressure is 760 torr. Using the formula $V_1/V_2 = P_2/P_1$, we get 100/x = 1140/760. x will equal 66.7 ml.

27. **(D)** When sublimation occurs, a substance changes directly from a solid to a gas without passing through a liquid phase.

28. **(A)** Acids always turn litmus paper red.

29. **(C)** Water is electrolyzed when it is placed in an electrical circuit. Electricity converts water to hydrogen (H_2) and oxygen (O_2). These two molecules can then be reconverted to water.

30. **(A)** pH is a measure of the H^+. When the H^+ is written as an exponent, the power of 10 is the negative pH. 0.001 m/1 can be written as 1×10^{-3}. Thus the solution has a pH of 3. A pH of less than 7 designates an acid.

31. **(D)** An electrolyte is a substance that conducts an electric current when added to water. To conduct a current, it must dissolve and carry an electrical charge. Only substances that are ionic *in solution* can be electrolytes.

32. **(D)** pH + pOH = 14. The OH^- concentration value is the negative of the exponent. Here pOH = 2. So 2 + pH = 14, and pH = 12.

33. **(A)** By definition, if the OH^- concentration is less than the H_3O^+ concentration, the solution is acidic. Acidic solutions have a pH less than 7.

34. **(B)** In a reduction reaction, electrons are gained. Al^{3+} represents aluminum with 13 protons and ten electrons. In choice B, when three electrons are added, aluminum is reduced and will have 13 protons and 13 electrons, and will be written simply as Al.

35. **(A)** For neutral molecules, oxidation numbers of all the atoms must add up to zero. The oxidation number is equal to the charge on the ion. In most

compounds containing oxygen, the oxidation number of each oxygen atom is 2–. In most compounds containing hydrogen, the oxidation number of each hydrogen atom is 1+.

36. (A) In this reaction, chlorine is being reduced (picking up electrons) and sodium is being oxidized (supplying electrons). So chlorine is the oxidizing agent (it is what is causing sodium to be oxidized) and sodium is the reducing agent (it is what is causing chlorine to be reduced).

37. (C) In a reduction reaction, electrons are gained and the oxidation number is reduced. Only in choice C is the oxidation number decreased.

38. (B) Catalysts change only the rate of a given reaction. They have no effects on the distribution of the products.

39. (D) Choices A, B, and C all increase the number of effective collisions between particles and thus speed up reactions.

40. (A) Sublimation occurs when a solid transforms directly to a gas without passing through a liquid phase. Entropy is a measure of disorder or randomness of a system. A gas has a less orderly arrangement of molecules than a solid. Thus when a solid turns into a gas, entropy increases.

41. (D) Higher equilibrium constants favor formation of products or the shift from left to right in any equation.

42. (D) Forms of the same element that differ only in neutron number are called isotopes. The atomic number (subscript before the element symbol) represents the number of protons in the atom. As atoms are electrically neutral, the number of electrons must equal the number of protons in the atom. The atomic weight of an atom is equal to the sum of the neutrons and protons.

43. (A) See explanation for question 42. Isotopes differ only in neutron number.

44. (B) Half-life denotes the time required for disintegration of $\frac{1}{2}$ of the atoms in a radioactive sample. After one half-life period, $\frac{1}{2}$ of a sample will remain, and after two half-life periods, $\frac{1}{2} \times \frac{1}{2}$ or $\frac{1}{4}$ of a sample will remain. Thus one hour must represent two half-life periods. The first half-life period must be half the hour.

45. (A) Alcohols are characterized by presence of a carbinol group: C - OH.

46. (A) This is acetaldehyde, an aldehyde. Aldehydes have a COH functional group where the carbon is double-bonded to the oxygen.

47. (B) Saturated hydrocarbons have the general formula C_nH_{2n+2}. Each carbon atom forms bonds to four other atoms, the maximum ("saturated") number of bonds possible for carbon.

48. (B) Esters result from the reaction of an organic acid with an alcohol. Esters always contain a carbon bonded to two oxygens.

49. (A) All choices are straight-chain saturated hydrocarbons with general formula C_nH_{2n+2}. The fewer carbons, the lower the boiling point. Methane, CH_4, has only one carbon.

50. (B) In fermentation, glucose breaks down to carbon dioxide and ethyl alcohol: $C_6H_{12}O_6 = CO_2 + C_2H_5OH$.

READING COMPREHENSION

1. **(D)** The author states (midway in the second paragraph) that the vagus nerve sends branches to specifically named organs. These organs are all concerned with vital involuntary functions. Therefore, it is suggested or implied that the vagus nerve is similarly concerned with involuntary regulation.

2. **(A)** All of the other choices are directly true of the vagus nerve and are stated in the passage. However, only the efferent fibers of the vagus nerve belong to the autonomic nervous system. This is verified near the end of the second paragraph.

3. **(D)** The second paragraph states that the heart is connected with the central nervous system by means of two nerves, the vagus and the cervical sympathetic. The last sentence in the first paragraph summarizes that the rate, force, and systolic output of the heart is controlled by nerves and by chemicals that nerve endings or other structures produce.

4. **(D)** This statement is made in the second sentence of the second paragraph, but not elaborated upon.

5. **(B)** The function of the heart is to discharge, with adequate force, an amount of blood sufficient for the metabolic needs of the body—that is, to pump blood. Impurities are cleared from the blood by the kidneys. Emotions have more effect upon the heart than the heart has upon emotions, despite popular misconception.

6. **(A)** White light contains rays of all colors. If all the light hitting a piece of cloth is reflected, then all the color rays will also be reflected. We will see all the color rays together as white.

7. **(B)** We can see only colors whose rays are reflected; if no rays are reflected, we can see only the absence of color, which is black.

8. **(C)** The word *translucent* comes from the Latin and means *to shine through*. If light is neither absorbed nor reflected, it must shine through. A translucent object may also be transparent, but light shining through does not automatically denote transparency. The object may diffuse the light which passes through so that objects beyond cannot be clearly distinguished.

9. **(B)** If the tie, which reflects only red light, were to have no red light waves to reflect, it would absorb all other colors and appear to be black.

10. **(A)** The only entirely true statement is that artificial light is different from sunlight. Incandescent light contains more red and yellow than sunlight, but other types of artificial light, fluorescent for example, do not. The transparency of glass has to do with its manufacture and with the way light is passed through the glass; it has nothing to do with the nature of the light that shines upon it.

11. **(C)** DNA, deoxyribonucleic acid, is a component of genes.

12. **(B)** An employer might find it very useful to screen prospective employees and to invest training time only in those who showed no genetic predisposition to diseases which might shorten the number of years of employment. But would such action be fair to an otherwise eager and able job candidate? This is as much a bioethical question as are those dealing with selective breeding.

13. **(D)** Bioengineering and genetic engineering refer to the manipulation of living genetic material.

14. **(A)** The application of the new genetic technology to disease control is projected for the future and is a most worthwhile goal, but, while research is in progress, the achievement itself is still in the ''possible'' category. As the third paragraph states, ''Researchers are not yet ready to predict a target date.''

15. **(D)** The subject is vast enough and important enough to be of concern to us all.

16. **(D)** Choices (A) and (C) are true statements but are only details, not the main idea, of the passage. There is no evidence to support answer (B). Choice (D) is the best expression of the main idea of the article and is also the hypothesis of the study.

17. **(A)** The basis of the Brookhaven study was to determine the extent of familial diseases and, in particular, high blood pressure. Choice (A), then, is the best answer. Although answers (B), (C), and (D) also seem correct, familial ties are not included in any of them, so they cannot be considered correct.

18. **(C)** Both the "R" and "S" strains of rats were injected with salt. It was each group's varying reaction to the salt that provided the main difference between the two groups. (C) is the correct answer.

19. **(C)** Sodium 22 does not cure or control high blood pressure; therefore, choices (A) and (D) are wrong. The "S" rats and the "R" rats were a known factor in the study, so answer (B) is also incorrect. The best answer is (C), and it is directly stated in the last sentence of the passage.

20. **(A)** Because the study was concerned with high blood pressure strains within families, this can lead to an early identification of the problem in family members, and preventive measures can be taken. This is most beneficial and best explained in answer (A), which is the correct answer. Answers (B) and (D) can be a result (thus secondary) of the early identification. Answer (C) is wrong, as the study did not lead to a cure.

21. **(D)** Paragraph two clearly states that "Other plants besides mint were tested and were found to have the same effect on the atmosphere."

22. **(C)** Notice that Priestley held this *belief* and used it as the *basis* for an experiment. By definition, then, his belief was a "hypothesis," a supposition or guess that is subjected to scientific testing. It couldn't be a "conclusion" (B) because he had not at that point performed the test that would provide a conclusion. It couldn't be an "analysis" (D) because he had not yet subjected the guess to any analytic process.

23. **(C)** Of the five choices, the "wheat field" (C) would have many many more plants than either "desert land" (A), a "cave" (B), or an "ice field" (D) and hence would have the "greater concentration of oxygen."

24. **(B)** The fourth sentence of paragraph two states outright that "the formation of oxygen occurred only in . . . sunlight" (B). This rules out independence from sunlight (A) and "any time of day," since night is without sun (C). Since the passage definitely says "only the green parts" produced oxygen, (D) is impossible.

25. **(A)** The author says, in paragraph two, that "in the process of adding oxygen to the air, plants simultaneously extracted another gaseous material, a substance we now know as carbon dioxide." (B), (C), and (D) are not mentioned directly in this connection.

26. **(D)** This is a good summary of the first two sentences.

27. **(C)** The only one of these conclusions supported by this study is (C). The statement is made in the last sentence of the first paragraph.

28. **(B)** The clue to this as the correct answer comes in the statement that man has a "much more efficient skin-ventilating system." (C) would be ridiculous because man is also "fed on proteins." (D) is wrong because it is the proteins that coagulate, not the blood. (A) may be true, but it is not cited as the ultimate cause of death.

29. **(B)** To coagulate is to change from a liquid to a more solid state. (A) is the exact opposite of the truth; (C) and (D) involve processes counter to coagulation.

30. (C) This inference is drawn from two facts: 1) it is a *skin*-ventilating system, and 2) skin is the body part closest, in other animals, to their fur.

31. (A) The paragraph deals with a specific mechanism and not with reproduction, the structure of DNA, or life's chemistry in general.

32. (D) DNA mediates protein synthesis through mRNA which it makes; therefore, (A) and (B) are incorrect. Transcription leads to translation, the assembly of amino acids into a protein structure, thereby making (D) correct.

33. (C) As defined in the passage, transcription is the process by which DNA makes mRNA.

34. (D) As stated in the passage, mRNA is a complement of DNA.

35. (B) This is stated and described in the first paragraph.

36. (D) The very first sentence in the passage states that this operation is the last resort for schizophrenia and manic-depression, both serious and advanced mental illnesses.

37. (B) The second sentence of the first paragraph describing the prefrontal lobotomy states that surgeons cut away important nerve connections in both the prefrontal brain lobe and thalamus.

38. (D) The last sentence of the first paragraph states that the operation's aim is to help the patient adjust better to the environment.

39. (B) The second paragraph describes the work of Dr. Walter R. Hess and his experiments with electrodes implanted in a cat's brain. The last sentence of that paragraph summarizes that Dr. Hess was able to determine how parts of the brain control organs of the body.

40. (C) The Nobel Prize in Medicine and Physiology was awarded jointly to Drs. Hess and Moniz.

41. (C) When carbon tetrachloride is added to pure bromine, the original red-brown color of the liquid changes to amber.

42. (D) A binary acid is one that contains only two elements, hydrogen and a nonmetal.

43. (A) An oxidizing agent reacts with metals, hydrogen, and water in its attempt to gain electrons to complete its outer shell.

44. (B) Hydrofluoric acid is instrumental in the production of cryolite. Cryolite, not the hydrofluoric acid itself, is used in the extraction of aluminum from its ore.

45. (C) The chemical activity of an element is governed by the number of electrons in its outer shell. Atoms are constantly striving to either gain or give up electrons. An element which strives to gain electrons serves as an oxidizing agent. The halogens, with their seven-electron shells, are searching to gain an eighth. Other oxidizing agents may have different numbers of electrons in their incomplete outer shells.

About the AHAT

• • • • • • • • • • • • • • •

The Allied Health Aptitude Test (AHAT) is a relatively new examination specifically designed for one- and two-year programs. It measures general academic ability and the scientific knowledge in the applicant's background. Currently 44 hospital schools and community colleges in the United States and three programs in Nova Scotia require that their applicants take this exam, and its acceptance is growing.

For the most part, the programs that require their applicants to take the AHAT arrange for its administration. There are only two scheduled testing centers: one in Dayton, Ohio, and the other in Johnstown, Pennsylvania. For more information about procedures for applying for this exam, you may contact the developer and administrator of the exam:

Allied Health Aptitude Test (AHAT)
The Psychological Corporation
55 Academic Court
San Antonio, TX 78204-3956
(512) 554-8200

The AHAT is a 280- to 300-question multiple-choice exam administered in four separately timed sections. The total testing time, including a short break between the second and third sections, is about three hours. All questions are equally weighted; that is, each is worth one point and there is no penalty for wrong answers. Separate raw scores (number right) and percentile rankings are reported for each of the four parts and for the exam as a whole.

The subjects of the AHAT are:

VERBAL ABILITY—approximately 90 questions in two styles

Directions: Choose the word that means the same or most nearly the same as the CAPITALIZED word.

1. ASPIRE
   1. Hope
   2. Breathe
   3. Exhaust
   4. Plot

2. FLAGRANT
   1. Disguised
   2. Glaring
   3. Repeated
   4. Perfumed

Directions: Choose the word that means the opposite or most nearly the opposite of the CAPITALIZED word.

3. DIMINISH

1. Lessen

2. Begin

3. Complete

4. Expand

4. SUCCUMB

1. Arrive

2. Yield

3. Eat

4. Conquer

NUMERICAL ABILITY—*approximately 60 questions in arithmetic, elementary algebra, and basic geometry*

Directions: Choose the best answer.

5. In its simplest form, $^{12}/_{16}$ is

1. $^3/_4$.

2. $^2/_3$.

3. $^2/_6$.

4. $^3/_8$.

6. If $y + 2 = 10$, then y must be

1. smaller than 10.

2. smaller than 8.

3. greater than 8.

4. equal to 0.

SCIENCE—*approximately 90 questions drawn from biology, chemistry, health, and the physical sciences*

Directions: Choose the best answer.

7. An eclipse of the sun throws the shadow of the

1. earth on the moon.

2. moon on the earth.

3. moon on the sun.

4. earth on the sun.

8. Light passes through the crystalline lens in the eye and focuses on the

1. cornea.

2. iris.

3. pupil.

4. retina.

READING SKILL—*approximately 40 questions based on reading passages on natural and social science topics*

Directions: Read the paragraph and answer the questions that follow on the basis of the information contained in the passage.

Using new tools and techniques, scientists, almost unnoticed, are remaking the world of plants. They have already remodeled 65 sorts of flowers, fruits, vegetables, and trees, giving us among other things tobacco that resists disease, cantaloupes that are immune to blight, and lettuce with crisper leaves. The chief new tool they are using is colchicine, a poisonous drug, which has astounding effects upon growth and upon heredity. It creates new varieties with astonishing frequency, whereas such mutations occur but rarely in nature. Colchicine has thrown new light on the fascinating jobs of the plant hunters. The Department of Agriculture sends people all over the world to find plants native to other lands that can be grown here and are superior to those already here. Scientists have crossed these foreign plants with those at home, thereby adding to our farm crops many desirable characteristics. The colchicine technique has enormously facilitated their work, because hybrids so often can be made fertile and because it takes so few generations of plants now to build a new variety with the qualities desired.

9. Colchicine speeds the improvement of plant species because it

   1. makes possible the use of foreign plants.
   2. makes use of natural mutations.
   3. creates new varieties very quickly.
   4. can be used with 65 different vegetables, fruits, and flowers.

10. Colchicine is a

    1. poisonous drug.
    2. technique.
    3. hybrid plant.
    4. blight.

ANSWERS: 1. 1　2. 2　3. 4　4. 4　5. 1
　　　　　6. 3　7. 2　8. 4　9. 3　10. 1

3

Information Sources

Professional Societies, Associations, and Boards

• • • • • • • • • • • • • •

The following is a listing of the societies, associations, and boards mentioned in the "For Additional Information" sections of the job descriptions, along with their addresses and telephone numbers for easy reference. There are also a number of other organizations listed that might be useful in obtaining information about other allied health careers.

Accrediting Bureau of Health Education Schools (ABHES)
29089 U.S. 20 West
Elkhart, IN 46514
(219) 293-0124

Alcohol and Drug Problems Association (ADPA)
444 North Capitol Street N.W.
Suite 181
Washington, DC 20001
(202) 737-4340

American Academy of Physician Assistants (AAPA)
1117 North 19th Street
Suite 300
Arlington, VA 22209
(703) 836-2272

American Association for Music Therapy (AAMT)
66 Morris Avenue
P.O. Box 359
Springfield, NJ 07081
(201) 379-1100

American Association for Clinical Chemistry (AACC)
1725 K Street N.W.
Suite 1010
Washington, DC 20006
(202) 857-0717

American Association for Counseling and Development (AACD)
5999 Stevenson Avenue
Alexandria, VA 22304
(703) 823-9800

American Association of Blood Banks (AABB)
1117 North 19th Street
Suite 600
Arlington, VA 22209
(703) 528-8200

American Association of Colleges of Pharmacy (AACP)
1426 Prince Street
Alexandria, VA 22314
(703) 739-2330

American Association of Colleges of Podiatric Medicine (AACPM)
6110 Executive Boulevard
Suite 204
Rockville, MD 20852
(301) 984-9350

American Association of Dental Examiners (AADE)
211 East Chicago Avenue
Suite 1812
Chicago, IL 60611
(312) 440-7464

American Association of Dental Schools (AADS)
1625 Massachusetts Avenue N.W.
Washington, DC 20036
(202) 667-9433

American Association of Homes for the Aging (AAHA)
1129 20th Street N.W.
Suite 400
Washington, DC 20036
(202) 783-2242

American Association of Medical Assistants (AAMA)
20 North Wacker Drive
Suite 1575
Chicago, IL 60606
(312) 692-7050

American Association of Nurse Anesthetists (AANA)
216 Higgins Road
Park Ridge, IL 60068
(312) 692-7050

American Association of Respiratory Care (AARC)
1720 Regal Row
Suite 112
Dallas, TX 75235
(214) 243-2272

American Board of Opticianry (ABO)
Opticians Association of America (OAA)
National Contact Lens Examiners (NCLE)
P.O. Box 10110
Fairfax, Virginia, 22030
(703) 691-8356

American Board of Registration for Electroencephalographic Technologists (ABRET)
University of California
Davis Medical Center
EEG Laboratory
2315 Stockton Boulevard
Sacramento, CA 95817
(916) 734-2011

American Chemical Society (ACS)
1155 16th Street N.W.
Washington, DC 20036
(202) 872-4600

American Chemical Society Career Services (ACSCS)
1155 16th Street N.W.
Washington, DC 20036
(202) 872-4600

American Chiropractic Association (ACA)
1701 Clarendon Boulevard
Arlington, VA 22909
(703) 276-8800

American College of Health Care Administrators (ACHCA)
8120 Woodmont Avenue
Suite 200
Bethesda, MD 20814
(301) 652-8384

American College of Healthcare Executives (ACHE)
840 North Lake Shore Drive
Suite 1103 W
Chicago, IL 60611
(312) 943-0544

American Council on Pharmaceutical Education (ACPE)
311 West Superior Street
Chicago, IL 60610
(312) 664-3575

American Dance Therapy Association (ADTA)
2000 Century Plaza
Suite 108
Columbia, MD 21044
(410) 997-4040

American Dental Assistants Association (ADAA)
666 North Lake Shore Drive
Suite 1130
Chicago, IL 60611
(312) 664-3327

American Dental Association (ADA)
211 East Chicago Avenue
Chicago, IL 60611
(312) 440-2500

American Dental Hygienists' Association (ADHA)
444 North Michigan Avenue
Suite 3400
Chicago, IL 60611
(312) 440-8900

American Dietetic Association (ADA)
216 West Jackson Boulevard
Suite 800
Chicago, IL 60606-6995
(312) 899-0040

American Geriatrics Society (AGS)
770 Lexington Avenue
New York, NY 10021
(212) 308-1414

American Health Care Association (AHCA)
1200 L Street N.W.
Washington, DC 20005
(202) 842-4444

American Hospital Association (AHA)
840 North Lake Shore Drive
Chicago, IL 60611
(312) 280-6000

American Institute of Biological Sciences (AIBS)
730 11th Street N.W.
Washington, DC 20001
(202) 628-1500

American Institute of Chemists (AIC)
7315 Wisconsin Avenue N.W.
Bethesda, MD 20814
(301) 652-2447

American Medical Association (AMA)
535 North Dearborn Street
Chicago, IL 60610
(312) 464-5000

American Medical Record Association (AMRA)
John Hancock Center
Suite 1850
875 North Michigan Avenue
Chicago, IL 60611
(312) 787-2672

American Medical Technologists (AMT)
710 Higgins Road
Park Ridge, IL 60068
(312) 823-5160

American Nurses' Association (ANA)
2420 Pershing Road
Kansas City, MO 64108
(816) 474-5720

American Occupational Therapy Association (AOTA)
P.O. Box 1725
1383 Piccard Drive
Rockville, MD 20850
(301) 948-9626

American Optometric Association (AOA)
243 North Lindbergh Boulevard
St. Louis, MO 63141
(314) 991-4100

American Physical Therapy Association (APTA)
1111 North Fairfax Street
Alexandria, VA 22314
(703) 684-2782

American Podiatric Medical Association (APMA)
9312 Old Georgetown Road
Bethesda, MD 20814
(301) 571-0920

American Registry of Clinical Radiography Technologists (ARCRT)
710 Higgins Road
Park Ridge, IL 60068
(312) 318-9050

American Registry of Diagnostic Medical Sonographers (ARDMS)
32 East Hollister Street
Cincinnati, OH 45219
(513) 721-6662

American Registry of Radiologic Technologists (ARRT)
1255 Northland Drive
Mendota Heights, MN 55120
(612) 687-0048

American Society of Aging (ASA)
833 Market Street
Suite 512
San Francisco, CA 94103
(415) 543-2617

American Society of Biological Chemists (ASBC)
9650 Rockville Pike
Bethesda, MD 20814
(301) 530-7145

American Society of Clinical Pathologists (ASCP)
2100 West Harrison
Chicago, IL 60612
(312) 738-1336

American Society of Cytology (ASC)
1015 Chestnut Street
Suite 1518
Philadelphia, PA 19107
(215) 922-3880

American Society of Electroneurodiagnostic Technologists (ASET)
204 West 7th
Carroll, IA 51401
(712) 792-2978

American Society of Hospital Pharmacists (ASHP)
4630 Montgomery Avenue
Bethesda, MD 20814
(301) 657-3000

American Society for Medical Technology (ASMT)
2021 L Street N.W.
Suite 400
Washington, DC 20036
(202) 785-3311

American Society of Radiologic Technologists (ASRT)
15000 Central Avenue S.E.
Albuquerque, NM 87123
(505) 298-4500

American Therapeutic Recreation Association (ATRA)
3101 Park Center Drive
Alexandria, VA 22302
(703) 820-4940
(800) 553-0304

American Veterinary Medical Association (AVMA)
930 North Meacham Road
Schaumburg, IL 60196
(312) 885-8070

Association for Gerontology in Higher Education (AGHE)
600 Maryland Avenue S.W.
Washington, DC 20024
(202) 484-7505

Association of Physician Assistant Programs (APAP)
950 North Washington Street
Alexandria, VA 22314
(703) 836-2272

Association of Schools and Colleges of Optometry (ASCO)
6110 Executive Boulevard
Rockville, MD 20852
(301) 231-5944

Association of Surgical Technologists (AST)
8307 Shaffer Parkway
Littleton, CO 80127
(303) 978-9010

Association of University Programs in Health Administration (AUPHA)
1911 Fort Myers Drive
Suite 503
Arlington, VA 22209
(703) 524-5500

Commission on Opticianry Accreditation (COA)
10111 M.L. King Jr. Hwy. #100
Bowie, MD 20720-4299
(301) 459-8075

Commission on Professionals in Science and Technology (CPST)
1500 Massachusetts Avenue N.W.
Suite 831
Washington, DC 29995
(202) 223-6995

Council on Chiropractic Education (CCE)
3209 Ingersoll Avenue
Des Moines, IA 50312
(515) 255-2184

Council on Social Work Education (CSWE)
1744 R Street N.W.
Washington, DC 20009
(202) 667-2300

Dental Assisting National Board, Inc. (DANB)
216 East Ontario Street
Chicago, IL 60611
(312) 642-3368

Division of Allied Health Education and Accreditation of the American Medical Association (DAHEAAMA)
535 North Dearborn Street
Chicago, IL 60610
(312) 464-4634

Gerontological Society of America (GSA)
1275 K Street N.W.
Washington, DC 20005
(202) 842-1275

International Chiropractors Association (ICA)
1901 L Street N.W.
Suite 800
Washington, DC 20036
(202) 659-6476

International Dance-Exercise Association (IDEA)
6190 Cornerstone St. E.
San Diego, CA 92121
(619) 535-8979

International Society for Clinical Laboratory Technology (ISCLT)
818 Olive Street
Suite 918
St. Louis, MO 63101
(314) 241-1445

Joint Review Committee for Respiratory Therapy Education (JRCRTE)
1701 West Euless Boulevard
Suite 200
Euless, TX 76040
(817) 283-2835

Joint Review Committee for the Accreditation of EEG Technology Training Programs (JRCFAETTP)
11526 53rd St. North
Clearwater, FL 34620

National Academy of Certified Clinical Mental Health Counselors (NACCMHC)
5999 Stevenson Avenue
Alexandria, VA 22304
(703) 823-9800

National Academy of Opticianry (NAO)
National Federation of Opticianry Schools (NFOS)
10111 M.L. King Jr. Hwy. #112
Bowie, Maryland 20720-4299
(301) 577-4828

National Association for Homecare (NAH)
519 C Street N.E.
Washington, DC 20002
(202) 547-7424

National Association for Music Therapy, Inc. (NAMT)
505 11th Street S.E.
Washington, DC 20003
(202) 543-6864

National Association for Practical Nurse Education and Service, Inc. (NAPNES)
1400 Spring Street
Suite 310
Silver Spring, MD 20910
(301) 588-2491

National Association of Activity Professionals (NAAP)
125 I Street N.W.
Washington, DC 20005
(202) 289-0722

National Association of Alcoholism and Drug Abuse Counselors (NAADAC)
3717 Columbia Pike
Suite 300
Arlington, VA 22204
(703) 920-4644

National Association of Boards of Pharmacy (NABP)
1300 Higgins Road
Suite 103
Park Ridge, IL 60068
(312) 698-6227

National Association of Emergency Medical Technicians (NAEMT)
9140 Ward Park
Kansas City, MO 64114
(816) 444-3500

National Association of Social Workers (NASW)
7981 Eastern Avenue
Silver Spring, MD 20910
(301) 565-0333

National Association of Substance Abuse Trainers and Educators (NASATE)
C/O Tom Lief
Substance Abuse Training Program
Southern University at New Orleans
6400 Press Drive
New Orleans, LA 70126
(504) 282-4401

National Board for Certified Counselors (NBCC)
5999 Stevenson Avenue
Alexandria, VA 22304
(703) 823-9800

National Board for Respiratory Care, Inc. (NBRC)
11015 West 75th Terrace
Shawnee Mission, KS 66214
(913) 268-4050

National Certification Agency for Medical Laboratory Personnel (NCAMLP)
1101 Connecticut Avenue N.W.
Suite 700
Washington, DC 20036
(202) 857-1100

National Clearinghouse on Alcoholism and Drug Abuse Information (NCADI)
P.O. Box 2345
Rockville, MD 20852
(301) 468-2600

National Commission on Certification of Physician Assistants, Inc. (NCCPA)
2845 Henderson Mill Road N.E.
Atlanta, GA 30341
(404) 493-9100

National Council for Therapeutic Recreation Certification (NCTRC)
49 South Main Street
Suite 5
Spring Valley, NY 10977
(914) 356-9660

National Federation of Licensed Practical Nurses, Inc. (NFLPN)
P.O. Box 1088
Raleigh, NC 27619
(919) 781-4791

National Health Council (NHC)
Health Careers Program
622 Third Avenue
New York, NY 10017
(212) 268-8900

National Institute on Drug Abuse (NIDA)
Office of Science
5600 Fishers Lane
Room 10-16
Rockville, MD 20857
(301) 443-6480

National Institutes of Health (NIH)
Division of Personnel Management
Bethesda, MD 20892
(301) 496-4197

National League for Nursing (NLN)
350 Hudson Street
New York, NY 10014
(212) 989-9393

National Registry of Emergency Medical Technicians
(614) 888-4484

National Society of Cardiovascular Technology/ National Society of Pulmonary Technology (NSCT/NSPT)
1133 15th Street N.W.
Suite 1000
Washington, DC 20005
(202) 371-1267

National Student Nurses' Association (NSNA)
555 West 57th Street
Suite 1325
New York, NY 10019
(212) 581-2211

National Therapeutic Recreation Society (NTRS)
3101 Park Center Drive
Alexandria, VA 22302
(703) 820-4940

Nuclear Medicine Technology Certification Board (NMTCB)
P.O. Box 806
Tucker, GA 30084
(404) 493-4504

Opticians Association of America (OAA)
10341 Democracy Lane
P.O. Box 10110
Fairfax, VA 22030
(703) 691-8355

Society of Diagnostic Medical Sonographers (SDMS)
12225 Greenville Avenue
Suite 435
Dallas, TX 75231
(214) 369-4332

**U.S. Office of Personnel Management
and the Veterans Administration (VA)**
1900 E Street N.W.
Washington, DC 20541
(202) 632-5491

Veterans Administration
810 Vermont Avenue N.W.
Washington, DC 20420
(202) 233-2741

Directory of Schools and Programs for the Twenty-Eight Representative Careers*

• • • • • • • • • • • • • •

PODIATRIST

(All programs approved by the American Association of Colleges of Podiatric Medicine)

California College of Podiatric Medicine
1210 Scott Street
P.O. Box 7855, Rincon Annex
San Francisco, CA 94120
(415) 563-8070

Barry University
11300 NE Second Avenue
Miami Shores, FL 33161
(305) 758-3392

Dr. William M. Scholl College
1001 North Dearborn Street
Chicago, IL 60610
(312) 567-3024

University of Osteopathic Medicine and Health Science
3200 Grand Avenue
Des Moines, IA 50312
(515) 271-1400

New York College of Podiatric Medicine
52 East 124th Street
New York, NY 10035
(212) 410-8000

Ohio College of Podiatric Medicine
10515 Carnegie Avenue
Cleveland, OH 44106
(216) 231-3300

Pennsylvania College of Podiatric Medicine
Eighth at Race Street
Philadelphia, PA 19107
(215) 923-6741

CHIROPRACTOR

(All programs accredited by the Council on Chiropractic Education)

Life Chiropractic College—West
2005 Via Barrett
San Lorenzo, CA 94580
(510) 276-9013

Palmer College of Chiropractic—West
1095 Dunford Way
Sunnyvale, CA 94087
(408) 983-4100

Life College
1269 Barclay Circle
Marietta, GA 30060
(404) 424-0554

* Listed alphabetically by states and within each state.

National College of Chiropractic
200 East Roosevelt Road
Lombard, IL 60148
(708) 629-9664

Palmer College of Chiropractic
1000 Brady Street
Davenport, IA 52803
(319) 326-9600

Northwestern College of Chiropractic
2501 West 84th Street
Bloomington, MN 55431
(612) 888-4777

Cleveland Chiropractic College
6401 Rockhill Road
Kansas City, MO 64131
(816) 333-8230

Logan College of Chiropractic
1851 Schoettler Road, POB 100
Chesterfield, MO 63017
(314) 227-2100

New York Chiropractic College
Route 89, P.O. Box 800
Seneca Falls, NY 13148
(315) 568-3000

Western States Chiropractic College
2900 Northeast 132nd Avenue
Portland, OR 97230
(503) 256-3180

Parker College of Chiropractic
300 E. Irving Boulevard
Irving, TX 75015
(214) 438-9355

Texas Chiropractic College
5912 Spencer Highway
Pasadena, TX 77505
(713) 487-1501

REGISTERED NURSE (R.N.)

Combined academic and clinical courses of study leading to the RN designation are offered by colleges, universities, and hospital schools throughout the country. Choice of location and the level of your previous background should lead you to the RN program which best suits your needs.

LICENSED PRACTICAL NURSE (LPN)

Since LPN's must complete a state-approved practical nursing program, you should contact your State Board of Nursing for its list of approved programs. Contact your State Board of Nursing at:

Alabama Board of Nursing
RSA Plaza, Suite 250
770 Washington Ave
Montgomery, AL 36130
(205) 242-4060

Alaska Board of Nursing
Department of Commerce & Economic Development
Div. of Occupational Licensing
3601 C Street, Suite 722
Anchorage, AK 99503

Arizona State Board of Nursing
2001 W. Camelback Road
Suite 350
Phoenix, AZ 85015

Arkansas State Board of Nursing
1123 South University
University Tower Bldg., Suite 800
Little Rock, AR 72204
(501) 371-2751

**California Board of Vocational Nurse
and Psychiatric Technician Examiners**
1414 K Street, Suite 103
Sacramento, CA 95814
(916) 445-0793

Colorado Board of Nursing
1560 Broadway, Suite 670
Denver, CO 80202
(303) 894-2430

Connecticut Board of Examiners for Nursing
150 Washington Street
Hartford, CT 06106
(203) 566-1041

Delaware Board of Nursing
Margaret O'Neill Bldg.
P.O. Box 1401
Dover, DE 19901
(302) 739-4522

District of Columbia Board of Nursing
614 H Street N.W.
Washington, D.C. 20001
(202) 727-7823
        7824

Florida Board of Nursing
111 Coastline Drive, East
Jacksonville, FL 32202
(904) 359-6331

Georgia State Board of Licensed Practical Nurses
166 Pryor Street, S.W.
Atlanta, GA 30303
(404) 656-3921

Hawaii Board of Nursing
P.O. Box 3469
Honolulu, HI 96801
(808) 586-2702

Idaho Board of Nursing
280 N. 8th Street, Suite 210
Boise, ID 83720
(208) 334-3110

Illinois Dept. of Registration and Education
320 West Washington Street
Third Floor
Springfield, IL 62786
(217) 785-0800

Indiana State Board of Nursing
Health Professions Bureau
One American Square
Suite 1020, Box 82067
Indianapolis, IN 46282-0004
(317) 232-2960

Iowa Board of Nursing
Executive Hills East
1223 East Court
Des Moines, IA 50319
(515) 281-3256

Kansas Board of Nursing
Landon State Office Bldg.
900 S.W. Jackson, Suite 551S
Topeka, KS 66612-1256
(913) 296-4929

Kentucky Board of Nursing
312 Whittington Parkway, Suite 300
Louisville, KY 40222-5172
(502) 329-7000

Louisiana State Board of Practical Nurse Examiners
Tidewater Place
1440 Canal Street, Suite 2010
New Orleans, LA 70112
(504) 568-6480

Maine State Board of Nursing
35 Anthony Street
State House Station #158
Augusta, ME 04333-0158

Maryland Board of Examiners of Nurses
4201 Patterson Avenue
Baltimore, MD 21215-2299
(410) 764-4747

Massachusetts Board of Registration in Nursing
Leverett Saltonstall Bldg.
100 Cambridge Street, Room 1519
Boston, MA 02202
(617) 727-7393

Michigan Board of Nursing
P.O. Box 30018
Lansing, MI 48909
(517) 373-1600

Minnesota Board of Nursing
2700 University Ave., W.
#108
St. Paul, MN 55114
(612) 642-0567

Mississippi Board of Nursing
239 N. Lamar Street
Suite 401
Jackson, MS 39201-1311
(601) 359-6170

Missouri State Board of Nursing
P.O. Box 656
3523 North Ten Mile Drive
Jefferson City, MO 65102
(314) 751-2334 Ext. 141

Montana State Board of Nursing
Dept. of Commerce
Division of Business and
Professional Licensing
1424 9th Avenue
Helena, MT 59620-0407
(406) 444-4279

Bureau of Examining Boards
Nebraska Dept. of Health
P.O. Box 95007
Lincoln, NE 68509
(402) 471-2115

Nevada State Board of Nursing
1281 Terminal Way
Suite 116
Reno, NV 89502
(702) 786-2778

New Hampshire Board of Nursing
Health & Welfare Building
6 Hazen Drive
Concord, NH 03301
(603) 271-2323

New Jersey Board of Nursing
1100 Raymond Boulevard
Suite 319
Newark, NJ 07102
(201) 648-2570

New Mexico Board of Nursing
4253 Montgomery N.E.
Suite 130
Albuquerque, NM 87109
(505) 841-8340

New York State Board for Nursing
State Education Department
Cultural Education Center
Room 9B30
Albany, NY 12230
(518) 474-3843

North Carolina Board of Nursing
P.O. Box 2129
Raleigh, NC 27602
(919) 782-3211

North Dakota Board of Nursing
919 South 7th Street
Suite 504
Bismarck, ND 58504
(710) 224-2974

Ohio Board of Nursing Education and Nurse Registration
65 South Front Street
Suite 509
Columbus, OH 43266-0316
(614) 466-3947

Oklahoma Board of Nurse Registration & Nursing Education
2915 N. Classen Boulevard
Suite 524
Oklahoma City, OK 73106
(405) 525-2076

Oregon State Board of Nursing
800 NE Oregon Street, #25
Portland, OR 97232
(503) 731-4745
FAX (503) 731-4755

Pennsylvania Board of Nursing
Department of State
P.O. Box 2649
Harrisburg, PA 17105
(717) 787-8503

Rhode Island Dept. of Health Professional Regulations
3 Capital Hill
Providence, RI 02908
(401) 277-2827

State Board of Nursing for South Carolina
220 Executive Center Drive
Suite 220
Columbia, SC 29210
(803) 737-6594

South Dakota Board of Nursing
3307 South Lincoln
Sioux Falls, SD 57105
(605) 335-4973

Tennessee State Board of Nursing
283 Plus Park Boulevard
Nashville, TN 37217
(615) 367-6232

Texas Board of Vocational Nurse Examiners
9101 Burnett Road
Suite 105
Austin, TX 78758
(512) 835-2071

Utah State Board of Nursing
Division of Occupational
& Professional Licensing
P.O. Box 45802
Salt Lake City, UT 84145
(801) 530-6733

Vermont State Board of Nursing
Redstone Building
26 Terrace Street
Montpelier, VT 05602

Virginia State Board of Nursing
1601 Rolling Hills Drive
Richmond, VA 23229-5005
(804) 662-9909

Washington State Board of Practical Nursing
P.O. Box 1099
Olympia, WA 98507
(206) 753-2807

**West Virginia State Board of Examiners
for Practical Nurses**
922 Quarrier Street
Embelton Bldg., Suite 506
Charleston, WV 25301
(304) 348-3572

Wisconsin Bureau of Health Professions
1400 East Washington Ave.
P.O. Box 8935
Madison, WI 53708-8935
(608) 266-3735

Wyoming State Board of Nursing
Barrett Building, 4th Floor
2301 Central Ave.
Cheyenne, WY 82002
(307) 777-7601

DENTAL HYGIENIST—DENTAL ASSISTANT

Over 375 institutions in all 50 states, the District of Columbia, and Puerto Rico offer educational programs accredited by the American Dental Association Commission on Dental Accreditation in either dental hygiene or dental assisting or both. There are well over 200 programs training dental hygienists and another 200-plus training dental assistants. In addition, the 26 programs in Canadian colleges that are approved by the Canadian Dental Association are recognized reciprocally. You can obtain a full list of the institutions that offer these programs (along with those offering programs in dental lab technology) and their mailing addresses by writing to:

American Dental Association
Commission on Dental Accreditation
211 East Chicago Avenue
Chicago, IL 60611
(312) 440-2500

ALCOHOL AND DRUG ABUSE COUNSELOR

There is no standardized, formal training program for becoming an alcohol and drug abuse counselor. Probably the majority of alcohol and drug abuse counselors come to the field by way of a Master of Social Work (MSW) degree, but the BA, BS, MA, MS, PhD, MEd, RN, and MD are all highly acceptable and common routes as well. Training in counseling can be gained on the job in highly structured and supervised settings, through in-service courses, and at workshops and seminars. Formal licensing is not required, but the National Association of Alcoholism and Drug Abuse Counselors (NAADAC) offers an examination and procedure leading to designation as a National Certified Addiction Counselor. This certification enhances employability and earning power.

DIETITIAN
(BA or BS degree programs approved by the American Dietetic Association)

Auburn University
Auburn University, AL 36849
(205) 844-4080

University of Alabama
Box UA
Tuscaloosa, AL 35487
(205) 348-5666

California State University, Los Angeles
5151 State University Drive
Los Angeles, CA 90032
(213) 343-3901

Loma Linda University
Loma Linda, CA 92350
(714) 785-2118

Saint Joseph College
1678 Asylum Avenue
West Hartford, CT 06117
(203) 232-4571 ext. 216

University of Connecticut
Storrs, CT 06268
(203) 486-3137

University of Delaware
Newark, DE 19716
(302) 451-8123

Howard University
2400 6th Street N.W.
Washington, DC 20059
(202) 686-6634

Florida International University
Tamiami Trail and 107th Avenue
Miami, FL 33177
(305) 554-3421

University of Florida
Gainesville, FL 32611
(904) 392-1365

Georgia State University
University Plaza
Atlanta, GA 30303-3085
(404) 651-2365

University of Idaho
Moscow, ID 83843
(208) 885-6326

Chicago State University
95th Street and King Drive
Chicago, IL 60628
(312) 995-2513

University of Illinois at Chicago
Box 5220
Chicago, IL 60680
(312) 996-0998

Indiana State University—Terre Haute
217 North 6th Street
Terre Haute, IN 47809
(812) 237-2121

Purdue University
West Lafayette, IN 47907
(317) 494-1776

Iowa State University of Science and Technology
Ames, IA 50011
(515) 294-5836

Kansas State University
Manhattan, KS 66506
(913) 532-6250

Spalding University
851 South 4th Street
Louisville, KY 40203
(502) 585-9911

University of Kentucky
100 W.D. Funkhouser Bldg.
Lexington, KY 40506-0054
(606) 257-2000

Hood College
Rosemont Avenue
Frederick, MD 21701-9988
(301) 663-3131 ext. 235

Framingham State College
100 State Street
Framingham, MA 01701
(508) 626-4500

Andrews University
Berrien Spring, MI 49104
(616) 471-3303

Eastern Michigan University
Ypsilanti, MI 48197
(313) 487-3060

Wayne State University
1142 Mackenzie Hall
Detroit, MI 48202
(313) 577-3577

College of Saint Benedict
College Avenue
Saint Joseph, MO 56374
(612) 363-5814

University of Minnesota, Twin Cities
231 Pillsbury Drive S.E.
240 Williamson Hall
Minneapolis, MN 55455
(612) 625-2008

University of Southern Mississippi
Southern Station Box 5011
Hattiesburg, MS 39406
(601) 266-5555

University of Missouri, Columbia
Columbia, MO 65211
(314) 882-7786

Rochester Institute of Technology
P.O. Box 9887
Rochester, NY 14623
(716) 475-5499

State University of New York at Buffalo
Buffalo, NY 14260
(716) 831-2111

Syracuse University
201 Tolley Administration Building
Syracuse, NY 13244
(315) 443-3611

North Dakota State University
University Station
Fargo, ND 58105
(701) 237-7752

University of North Dakota
Box 8095 University Station
Grand Forks, ND 58202
(701) 777-2711

Ohio State University
1800 Cannon Drive
Columbus, OH 43210
(614) 292-3980

University of Akron
302 Buchtel Commons
Akron, OH 44325
(216) 972-7100

University of Oklahoma
660 Parrington Oval
Norman, OK 73019
(405) 325-2251

Edinboro University of Pennsylvania
Edinboro, PA 16444
(814) 732-2720

Immaculata College
Immaculata, PA 19345
(215) 296-9067

Marywood College
2300 Adams Avenue
Scranton, PA 18509
(717) 348-6234

Mercyhurst College
501 East 38th Street
Erie, PA 16546
(814) 825-0240

Seton Hill College
Greensburg, PA 15601
(412) 838-4255

University of Pittsburgh
Second Floor, Bruce Hall
Pittsburgh, PA 15260
(412) 624-7488

Pan American University
1201 W. University Drive
Edinburg, TX 78539
(512) 381-2011

Texas Christian University
2800 South University Drive
Forth Worth, TX 76129
(817) 921-7490

University of Texas, Austin
University Station
Austin, TX 78712-1159
(512) 471-1711

University of Texas, Health Science Center at Houston
P.O. Box 20036
Houston, TX 77225
(713) 792-4975

University of Texas, Southwestern Medical Center at Dallas
5323 Henry Hines Boulevard
Dallas, TX 75235
(214) 688-3404

Brigham Young University
Provo, UT 84602
(801) 378-2507

Utah State University
Logan, UT 84322
(801) 750-1006

Virginia Polytechnic Institute and State University
Blacksburg, VA 24061
(703) 321-6267

Eastern Washington University
M.S. 148 Admissions Office
Cheney, WA 99004
(509) 359-2397

Washington State University
342 French Administration
Pullman, WA 99164
(509) 335-5586

University of Wisconsin, Madison
500 Lincoln Drive
Madison, WI 53706
(608) 262-3961

Viterbo College
815 South 9th Street
La Crosse, WI 54601
(608) 784-0040

EEG TECHNOLOGIST/TECHNICIAN

(Recognized schools for Electroneurodiagnostic Technology. Those marked * are accredited by the Committee on Allied Health Education Accreditation of the American Medical Association.)

*Barrow Neurological Institute of St. Joseph's Hospital and Medical Center
P.O. Box 2071
Phoenix, AZ 85001
(602) 285-3278
24-month program leading to AAS degree

*Orange Coast College
Neurodiagnostic Technologist Program
2701 Fairview Road
P.O. Box 5005
Costa Mesa, CA 92628-0120
(714) 432-5591
18-month program leading to AA degree

*St. Joseph's Hospital
School of EEG Technology
P.O. Box 4227
3001 Dr. Martin Luther King Jr. Boulevard
Tampa, FL 33677
(813) 870-4453—EEG Lab
15-month program leading to diploma

Shands Hospital at the University of Florida
Box 100365, Neurologic Functions
Neurodiagnostic Training Program
Gainesville, FL 32610
(904) 395-0334
12-month program leading to certificate

Medical College of Georgia
Department of Neurology
Augusta, GA 30912
(404) 721-4512
8 quarters leading to AS degree

East-West University
ENDT Program
816 S. Michigan Avenue
Chicago, IL 60605
(312) 939-0111
18-month program leading to AAS degree

*St. John's Hospital
Electroencephalographic Tech Program
800 East Carpenter Street
Springfield, IL 62769
(217) 544-6464, ext. 4704
12-month program leading to diploma

Kirkwood Community College of Cedar Rapids, IA
Electroencephalography Technology Program
University of Iowa Hospital
1084 Carver Pavilion
Iowa City, IA 52242
(319) 356-8766
21-month program leading to AAS degree

Scott Community College
Neurodiagnostic Technology Program
500 Bellmont Ed
Bettendorf, IA 52722
(319) 359-7531
24-month program leading to AAS degree

*Naval School of Health Sciences
Electroneurodiagnostic Technician Program
8901 Wisconsin Avenue
Bethesda, MD 20889-5033
(301) 295-0214
6-month program leading to certificate

*Children's Hospital Medical Center
Electroencephalographic Technology Program
300 Longwood Avenue
Boston, MA 02115
(617) 735-7970
12-month program leading to certificate

*Catherine Labouré College
Clinical Neurophysiology Technology
2120 Dorchester Avenue
Boston, MA 02124
(617) 296-8300, ext. 4043
20-month program leading to AS degree

*Anoka-Hennepin Vocational Technical School
Electroencephalographic Technologist Program
1355 W. Highway 10
Anoka, MN 55303
(612) 427-1880
12-month program leading to diploma; 18-month program leading to AAS degree

Mayo Medical Center
Clinical Neurophysiology Technology Program
Damon 53
Rochester, MN 55905
(507) 284-1255
24-month program leading to AAS degree

*Niagara County Community College
Electroneurodiagonistic Technologist Program
3111 Saunders Settlement Road
Sandborn, NY 14132
(716) 731-3271
20-month program leading to AAS degree

Southwestern Community College
275 Webster Road
Sylva, NC 28779
(704) 586-4091
12-month program leading to diploma

Carlow College
School of EEG at Children's Hospital of Pittsburgh
3705 5th Avenue
Pittsburgh, PA 15213
(412) 692-6164
15-month program leading to certificate

*Crozier-Chester Medical Center
School of EEG
15th and Upland Avenue
Chester, PA 19013
(215) 447-2688
12-month program leading to certificate

*Sentara Norfolk General Hospital
School of EEG Technology
600 Gresham Avenue
Norfolk, VA 23507
(804) 628-4240
18-month program leading to certificate

*Western Wisconsin Technical Institute
EEG Technology Program
304 N. 6th Street, P.O. Box 908
LaCrosse, WI 54602
(608) 785-6253
20-month program leading to AAS degree

British Columbia Institute of Technology
3700 Willingdon Avenue
Burnaby, BC, Canada V5G 3H2
(604) 432-8664
2-year program leading to diploma of technology

EKG TECHNICIAN

Formal, standardized training programs for EKG (electrocardiogram) technicians are located in hospital schools, community colleges, and independent allied health technical schools throughout the country. Large medical practices and clinics offer less formal, hands-on training programs. It is possible to start with less sophisticated on-the-job training and later to advance by taking courses in more complex procedures and in interpretation of readings.

EMERGENCY MEDICAL TECHNICIAN

(Certificate or degree programs approved by Council on Medical Education of the American Medical Association and the American College of Emergency Physicians, American College of Surgeons, American Society of Anesthesiologists, National Association of Medical Technicians, and National Registry of Emergency Medical Technicians)

Gadsden State Community College
P.O. Box 227
Gadsden, AL 35999-0277
(205) 546-0484

George C. Wallace State Community College
Dothan, AL 36303
(205) 983-3521

University of Alabama at Birmingham
University Station
Birmingham, AL 35294
(205) 934-8221

University of Alabama in Huntsville
Huntsville, AL 35899
(205) 895-6070

Central Arizona College
Woodruff at Overfield Road
Coolidge, AZ 85228
(602) 836-8243

Crafton Hills College
11711 Sand Canyon Road
Yucaipa, CA 92399
(714) 794-2161

Arapahoe Community College
2500 W. College Drive
Littleton, CO 80120-1955
(303) 794-1550

University of Colorado Health Sciences Center
4200 East 9th Avenue
Denver, CO 80262
(303) 399-1211

Brevard Community College
1519 Clearlake Road
Cocoa, FL 32922
(407) 632-1111

Broward Community College
225 East Las Olas Boulevard
Fort Lauderdale, FL 33301
(305) 475-6500

Central Florida Community College
P.O. Box 1388
Ocala, FL 32678
(904) 237-2111

Daytona Beach Community College
Box 1111
Daytona Beach, FL 32015
(904) 255-8131

Edison Community College
8099 College Parkway, SW
Fort Myers, FL 33906
(813) 489-9300

Florida Community College at Jacksonville
501 West State Street
Jacksonville, FL 32202
(904) 632-3000

Gulf Coast Community College
5230 West Highway 98
Panama City, FL 32401
(904) 769-1551

Hillsborough Community College
P.O. Box 31127
Tampa, FL 33631
(813) 253-7000

Indian River Community College
3209 Virginia Avenue
Fort Pierce, FL 33454
(407) 468-4700

Lake City Community College
Route 3, Box 7
Lake City, FL 32055
(904) 752-1822

Miami-Dade Community College
300 N.E. Second Avenue
Miami, FL 33132
(305) 347-1000

Palm Beach Community College
4200 Congress Avenue
Lake Worth, FL 33461
(407) 439-8000

Pasco-Hernando Community College
2401 State Highway 41 North
Dade City, FL 33525
(904) 567-6701

Pensacola Junior College
1000 College Boulevard
Pensacola, FL 32504
(904) 484-1000

Polk Community College
999 Avenue H, N.E.
Winter Haven, FL 33881
(813) 294-7771

Santa Fe Community College
3000 Northwest 83rd Street
P.O. Box 1530
Gainesville, FL 32602
(904) 395-5443

St. Petersburg Junior College
8580 66th Street North
Pinellas Park, FL 24665-1207
(813) 341-3600

Tallahassee Community College
444 Appleyard Drive
Tallahassee, FL 32304-2895
(904) 488-9200

Valencia Community College
P.O. Box 3028
Orlando, FL 32802
(407) 299-5000

Johnson County Community College
12345 College Boulevard
Overland Park, KS 66201
(913) 469-8500

Eastern Kentucky University
Lancaster Avenue
Richmond, KY 40475
(606) 622-2106

Northeast Metro Tech Institute
3300 Century Avenue, N.
White Bear Lake, MN 55110
(612) 770-2351

Creighton University
2500 California Street
Omaha, NE 68178
(402) 280-2703

New Hampshire Technical Institute
P.O. Box 2039
Concord, NH 03301
(603) 225-1800

University of New Mexico
Albuquerque, NM 87131
(505) 277-2446

Catawba Valley Community College
Route 3, Box 283
Hickory, NC 28602
(704) 327-9124

Western Carolina University
Cullowhee, NC 28723
(704) 227-7317

Columbus State Community College
P.O. Box 1609
Columbus, OH 43216
(614) 227-2400

Youngstown State University
410 Wick Avenue
Youngstown, OH 44555
(216) 742-3150

Portland Community College
12000 Southwest 49th Avenue
Portland, OR 97219
(503) 244-6111

Greenville Technical College
P.O. Box 5616, Station B
Greenville, SC 29606
(803) 250-8000

Jackson State Community College
2046 North Parkway Street
Jackson, TN 38301
(901) 424-3520

Roane State Community College
Patton Lane
Harriman, TN 37748
(615) 354-3000

Shelby State Community College
Box 40568
Memphis, TN 38174-0568
(901) 528-6700

Volunteer State Community College
Nashville Pike
Gallatin, TN 37066
(615) 452-8600

Austin Community College
P.O. Box 2285
Austin, TX 78768
(512) 488-7000

Texas Tech University
P.O. Box 4049
Lubbock, TX 79409
(806) 742-3652

University of Texas Health Science Center at San Antonio
7703 Floyd Curl Drive
San Antonio, TX 78284
(512) 567-2621

University of Texas Southwestern Medical Center at Dallas
5323 Henry Hines Boulevard
Dallas, TX 75235
(214) 688-3404

Northern Virginia Community College
8333 Little River Turnpike
Annandale, VA 22003
(703) 323-3000

Central Washington University
Ellensburg, WA 98926
(509) 963-1211

Spokane Community College
North 1810 Greene Street
Spokane, WA 99207
(509) 536-7000

Tacoma Community College
5900 South 12th Street
Tacoma, WA 98465
(206) 566-5000

University of Washington
1400 Northeast Campus Parkway
Seattle, WA 98195
(206) 543-9686

Medical College of Wisconsin
8701 Watertown Plank Road
Milwaukee, WI 53226
(414) 257-8246

MEDICAL RECORDS TECHNICIAN
(All programs accredited by the Council on Medical Education of the American Medical Association and the American Medical Record Association.)

University of Alabama at Birmingham
University Station
Birmingham, AL 35294
(205) 934-8221

Phoenix College
1202 West Thomas Road
Phoenix, AZ 85013
(602) 264-2492

Chabot College
25555 Hesperian Boulevard
Hayward, CA 94545
(415) 786-6600

City College of San Francisco
50 Phelan Avenue
San Francisco, CA 94112
(415) 239-3000

Cypress College
9200 Valley View Street
Cypress, CA 90630
(714) 826-2220

East Los Angeles College
1301 West Brooklyn Avenue
Monterey Park, CA 91754
(213) 265-8650

San Diego Mesa College
7250 Mesa College Drive
San Diego, CA 92111
(619) 560-2600

Arapahoe Community College
2500 West College Drive
Littleton, CO 80120
(303) 794-1550

Briarwood College
2279 Mount Vernon Road
Southington, CT 06489
(203) 628-4751

Daytona Beach Community College
1200 Volusia Avenue
Daytona Beach, FL 32114
(904) 255-8131

Miami-Dade Community College
300 N.E. Second Avenue
Miami, FL 33132
(305) 347-1000

Pensacola Junior College
1000 College Boulevard
Pensacola, FL 32504
(904) 484-1000

St. Petersburg Junior College
8580 66th Street North
Pinellas Park, FL 34666
(813) 341-3600

Boise State University
1910 University Drive
Boise, ID 83725
(208) 385-1156

Belleville Area College
2500 Carlyle Road
Belleville, IL 62221
(618) 235-2700

College of Dupage
22nd Street and Lambert Road
Glen Ellyn, IL 60137
(708) 858-2800

College of Lake County
19351 West Washington Street
Grayslake, IL 60030
(708) 223-6601

Harry S Truman College, City Colleges of Chicago
1145 Wilson Avenue
Chicago, IL 60640
(312) 878-1700

Moraine Valley Community College
10900 South 88th Avenue
Palos Hills, IL 60495
(708) 974-4300

Oakton Community College
1600 East Golf Road
Des Plaines, IL 60016
(708) 635-1600

Indiana University Northwest
3400 Broadway
Gary, IN 46408
(219) 980-6821

Vincennes University
1002 North First Street
Vincennes, IN 47591
(812) 885-4313

Indian Hills Community College
721 North First Street
Centerville, IA 52544
(515) 856-2143

Kirkwood Community College
6301 Kirkwood Boulevard, S.W.
Cedar Rapids, IA 52406
(319) 398-5411

Dodge City Community College
2501 North 14th Avenue
Dodge City, KS 67801
(316) 225-1321

Washburn University of Topeka
1700 College
Topeka, KS 66621
(913) 295-6625

Eastern Kentucky University
Lancaster Avenue
Richmond, KY 40475
(606) 622-2106

Western Kentucky University
College Heights
Bowling Green, KY 42101
(502) 745-2551

Louisiana Tech University
P.O. Box 3186 Tech Station
Ruston, LA 71272
(318) 257-3036

University of Maine at Bangor
Lincoln Hall
Bangor, ME 04401

Community College of Baltimore, Liberty Campus
2901 Liberty Heights Avenue
Baltimore, MD 21215
(410) 396-0203

Prince George's Community College
301 Largo Road
Largo, MD 20772
(301) 336-6000

Holyoke Community College
303 Homestead Avenue
Holyoke, MA 01040
(413) 538-7000

Laboure College
2120 Dorchester Avenue
Boston, MA 02124
(617) 296-8300, ext. 4005

Massachusetts Bay Community College
50 Oakland Street
Wellesley, MA 02181
(617) 237-1100

Northern Essex Community College
100 Elliott Street
Haverhill, MA 01830
(508) 374-3900

Cleary College
2170 Washtenaw Avenue
Ypsilanti, MI 48197
(313) 483-4400

Ferris State University
Big Rapids, MI 49307
(616) 592-2100

Henry Ford Community College
5101 Evergreen Road
Dearborn, MI 48128
(313) 271-2750

Mercy College of Detroit
8200 West Outer Drive
Detroit, MI 48219
(313) 592-6030

Muskegon Community College
221 South Quarterline Road
Muskegon, MI 49442
(616) 773-9131

Schoolcraft College
18600 Haggerty Road
Livonia, MI 48152
(313) 591-6400

Anoka Area Voc Tech Institute
1355 West Main Street, Box 191
Anoka, MN 55303
(612) 427-1880

College of Saint Catherine
2004 Randolph Street
St. Paul, MN 55105
(612) 690-6505

Moorhead Technical College
1900 28th Avenue South
Moorhead, MN 56560
(218) 236-6277

Hinds Community College
Raymond, MS 39154
(601) 857-5261

Meridian Community College
5500 Highway 19 North
Meridian, MS 39305
(601) 483-8241

Penn Valley Community College
3201 Southwest Trafficway
Kansas City, MO 64111
(816) 932-7600

College of Saint Mary
1901 South 72nd Street
Omaha, NE 68124
(402) 399-2405

New Hampshire Vocational-Technical College
Hanover Street Extension
Claremont, NH 03743
(603) 542-7744

Hudson County Community College
168 Sip Avenue
Jersey City, NJ 07306
(201) 656-2020

Union County College
1033 Springfield Avenue
Cranford, NJ 07016
(908) 709-7000

Broome Community College
Upper Front Street, Box 1017
Binghamton, NY 13902
(607) 771-5000

Manhattan Community College (CUNY)
199 Chambers Street

New York, NY 10007
(212) 618-1222

Mohawk Valley Community College
1101 Sherman Drive
Utica, NY 13501
(315) 792-5354

Monroe Community College
1000 East Henrietta Road
Rochester, NY 14623
(716) 424-5200

Onondaga Community College
Syracuse, NY 13215
(315) 469-7741

Rochester Institute of Technology
P.O. Box 9887
Rochester, NY 14623
(716) 475-5499

Rockland Community College
145 College Road
Suffern, NY 10901
(914) 356-4650

State University of New York College of Technology at Alfred
Alfred, NY 14802
(607) 587-4215

Central Piedmont Community College
Box 35009
Charlotte, NC 28235
(704) 342-6633

North Dakota State College of Science
Wahpeton, ND 58075
(701) 671-2201

Bowling Green State University
Bowling Green, OH 43404
(419) 372-2086

Cincinnati Technical College
3520 Central Parkway
Cincinnati, OH 45223
(513) 569-1500

Cuyahoga Community College
700 Carnegie Avenue
Cleveland, OH 44115
(216) 987-4000

Sinclair Community College
444 West Third Street
Dayton, OH 45402
(513) 226-2500

Stark Technical College
6200 Frank Avenue, N.W.
Canton, OH 44720
(216) 494-6170

Central Oregon Community College
2600 N.W. College Way
Bend, OR 97701
(503) 385-5500

Portland Community College
12000 Southwest 49th Avenue
Portland, OR 97219
(503) 244-6111

Community College of Allegheny County, Allegheny Campus
808 Ridge Avenue
Pittsburgh, PA 15212
(412) 237-2525

Community College of Philadelphia
17th and Spring Garden Streets
Philadelphia, PA 19130
(215) 751-8000

Gwynedd-Mercy College
Gwynedd Valley, PA 19437
(215) 641-5510

South Hills Business School
480 Waupilini Drive
State College, PA 16801
(814) 234-7755

Puerto Rico Junior College
Munoz Rivera Esq. Universidad
Rio Piedras, PR 00928
(809) 758-7171

Midlands Technical College
316 South Beltline Boulevard
Columbia, SC 29205
(803) 738-1400

Dakota State College
Heston Hall
Madison, SD 57042
(605) 256-5139

Chattanooga State Technical Community College
4501 Amnicola Highway
Chattanooga, TN 37406
(615) 697-4400

Roane State Community College
Patton Lane
Harriman, TN 37748
(615) 354-3000

Volunteer State Community College
Nashville Pike
Gallatin, TN 37066
(615) 452-8600

El Paso Community College
P.O. Box 20500
El Paso, TX 79998
(915) 594-2000

South Plains College
1401 College Avenue
Levelland, TX 79336
(806) 894-9611

St. Philip's College
211 Nevada Street
San Antonio, TX 78203
(512) 531-3200

Tarrant County Junior College
1500 Houston Street
Fort Worth, TX 76102-6599
(817) 336-7851

Texas State Technical Institute, Harlingen Campus
Box 2628
Harlingen, TX 78551
(512) 425-4922

Wharton County Junior College
911 Boling Highway
Wharton, TX 77488
(409) 532-4560

Weber State College
Ogden, UT 84408
(801) 626-6050

Central Virginia Community College
3506 Wards Road South
Lynchburg, VA 24502
(804) 386-4500

Northern Virginia Community College
8333 Little River Turnpike
Annandale, VA 22003
(703) 323-3000

Tidewater Community College
State Route 135
Portsmouth, VA 23703
(804) 484-2121

Shoreline Community College
16101 Greenwood Avenue N.
Seattle, WA 98133
(205) 546-4101

Spokane Community College
North 1810 Greene Street
Spokane, WA 99207
(509) 536-7000

Tacoma Community College
5900 South 12th Street
Tacoma, WA 98465
(206) 566-5000

Fairmont State College
Fairmont, WV 26554
(304) 367-4141

Marshall University
400 Hal Greer Boulevard
Huntington, WV 25755
(304) 696-3160

Chippewa Valley Technical College
620 West Clairmont Avenue
Eau Claire, WI 54701
(715) 833-6200

Moraine Park Technical College
235 North National Avenue
Fond du Lac, WI 54935
(414) 922-8611

Western Wisconsin Technical College
304 Sixth Street North
LaCrosse, WI 54601
(608) 785-9200

PHYSICIAN ASSISTANT

*(Degree and certificate programs at institutions accred-
ited by the American Medical Association in collaboration with the American Academy of Family Physicians,
the American Academy of Pediatrics, American Academy of Physician Assistants, American College of Physicians, American College of Surgeons, and the
Association of Physician Assistant Programs.)*

Stanford University
Stanford, CA 94305
(415) 723-2091

University of California, Davis
Davis, CA 95616
(916) 752-2971

University of Southern California
SAS 342-University Park
Los Angeles, CA 90089-0911
(213) 743-6741

University of Colorado at Denver
1200 Larimer Street
Denver, CO 80204-5300
(303) 556-2275

Yale University
1502A Yale Station
New Haven, CT 06520
(203) 432-1900

George Washington University
Washington, DC 20052
(202) 994-6040

Howard University
2400 6th Street N.W.
Washington, DC 20059
(202) 686-6634

University of Florida
Gainesville, FL 32611
(904) 392-1365

Emory University
Atlanta, GA 30322
(404) 727-6036

Medical College of Georgia
1120 15th Street
Augusta, GA 30912
(404) 721-2725

Chicago City-Wide College
226 West Jackson Boulevard
Chicago, IL 60606
(312) 641-2595

University of Iowa
Iowa City, IA 52242
(319) 335-3847

University of Osteopathic Medicine and Health Sciences
3200 Grand Avenue
Des Moines, IA 50312
(515) 271-1400

Wichita State University
1845 Fairmount
Wichita, KS 67208
(316) 689-3085

University of Kentucky
100 W.D. Funkhouser Bldg.
Lexington, KY 40506-0054
(606) 257-2000

Essex Community College
7201 Rossville Boulevard
Baltimore County, MD 21237
(410) 682-6000

Northeastern University
360 Huntington Avenue
Boston, MA 02115
(617) 437-2200

Mercy College of Detroit
8200 West Outer Drive
Detroit, MI 48219
(313) 592-6030

Western Michigan University
Kalamazoo, MI 49008
(616) 383-1950

Saint Louis University
221 North Grand Boulevard
St. Louis, MO 63103
(314) 658-2500

University of Nebraska at Omaha
Omaha, NE 68182
(402) 554-2393

New Jersey University of Medicine and Dentistry
150 Bergen Street
Newark, NJ 07103-2406
(201) 456-4300

State University of New York at Stony Brook
Stony Brook, NY 11794
(516) 632-6868

Touro College
844 Avenue of the Americas
New York, NY 10001-4103
(212) 447-0700

Duke University
2138 Campus Drive
Durham, NC 27706
(919) 684-3214

University of North Dakota
Box 8095, University Station
Grand Forks, ND 58202
(701) 777-2711

Cuyahoga Community College
700 Carnegie Avenue
Cleveland, OH 44115
(216) 987-4000

Kettering College of Medical Arts
3737 Southern Boulevard
Kettering, OH 45429
(513) 296-7201

University of Oklahoma Medical Center
P.O. Box 2690
Oklahoma City, OK 73190
(405) 271-2265

Gannon University
University Square
Erie, PA 16541
(814) 871-7240

Hahnemann University/School of Health Sciences
201 North 15th Street
Mail Stop 506
Philadelphia, PA 19102-1192
(215) 448-8288

King's College
133 N. River Street
Wilkes-Barre, PA 18711
(717) 826-5858

Saint Francis College
Loretto, PA 15940
(814) 472-3100

Trevecca Nazarene College
333 Murfreesboro Road
Nashville, TN 37203
(615) 248-1200

Baylor College of Medicine
One Baylor Plaza
Houston, TX 77030
(713) 798-4841

University of Texas Medical Branch
541 Administration Building
300 University Boulevard
Galveston, TX 77550
(409) 761-1011

University of Texas Southwestern Medical Center at Dallas
5323 Henry Hines Boulevard
Dallas, TX 75235
(214) 688-3111

University of Utah
Salt Lake City, UT 84112
(801) 581-7281

University of Washington
1400 Northeast Campus Parkway
Seattle, WA 98195
(206) 543-9686

Alderson-Broaddus College
Philippi, WV 26416
(304) 457-1700

University of Wisconsin, Madison
500 Lincoln Drive
Madison, WI 53706
(608) 262-3961

CLINICAL LABORATORY TECHNOLOGIST

There are over 200 degree programs in medical technology in Schools of Medical Technology that are approved by the American Medical Association's Council on Medical Education in cooperation with the American Society of Clinical Pathologists and American Society for Medical Technology. These programs may be found in major colleges and universities throughout the United States and Puerto Rico. There are also over 300 associate degree programs for Medical Laboratory Technicians approved by the National Accrediting Agency for Clinical Laboratory Sciences and the American Medical Association in collaboration with the American Society of Clinical Pathologists and the American Society of Medical Technology. These programs may be found in community and technical colleges as well as in four-year colleges. In addition, there are a number of training programs for specialties within the clinical laboratory technician/technologist field.

Blood Bank Technology: 15 degree or certificate programs approved by the Council on Medical Education of the American Medical Association in collaboration with the American Association of Blood Banks.

Cytotechnology: 60 degree or certificate programs approved by the Council on Medical Education of the American Medical Association in collaboration with the American Society of Cytology.

Histologic Technology: 20 certificate or degree programs approved by the Council on Medical Education of the American Medical Association in collaboration with the American Society of Clinical Pathologists, the

American Society of Medical Technologists, and the National Society for Histotechnology.

HEALTH SERVICES ADMINISTRATOR

According to the Association of University Programs in Health Administration (AUPHA), there are currently 87 undergraduate degree programs in health services administration. 55 of these programs offer an accredited master's program as well. The master's program in Health Services Administration are approved by the Accrediting Commission on Education for Health Services Administration (ACEHSA). Only seven of the undergraduate programs are accredited by AUPHA. In all of these, the graduate programs are accredited by ACEHSA as well. The seven approved undergraduate programs are:

Governors State University
University Park, IL 60466
(312) 534-5000, ext. 2511

University of Kentucky
100 W.D. Funkhouser Bldg.
Lexington, KY 40506-0054
(606) 257-2000

University of North Carolina at Chapel Hill
Chapel Hill, NC 27514
(919) 966-3621

Pennsylvania State University
201 Shields Building
University Park, PA 16802
(814) 865-5471

Meharry Medical College
1005 Dr. D. B. Todd Boulevard
Nashville, TN 37208
(615) 237-6000

Southwest Texas State University
San Marcos, TX 78666
(512) 245-2364

Virginia Commonwealth University
910 West Franklin Street, Box 2526
Richmond, VA 23284
(804) 257-6124

A master's degree in health services administration accredited by the Accrediting Commission on Education For Health Services Administration can also be earned at the following universities:

University of Alabama at Birmingham
University Station
Birmingham, AL 35294
(205) 934-8221

Arizona State University
Tempe, AZ 85287
(602) 965-7788

University of Arkansas at Little Rock
2801 South University
Little Rock, AR 72204
(501) 569-3127

San Diego State University
5402 College Avenue
San Diego, CA 98182-0771
(619) 594-5384

University of California, Berkeley
Berkeley, CA 94720
(415) 642-2949

University of California, Los Angeles
405 Hilgard Avenue
Los Angeles, CA 90024
(213) 825-3101

University of Southern California
SAS 342-University Park
Los Angeles, CA 90089-0911
(213) 743-6741

University of Denver
University Park
Denver, CO 80208
(303) 871-2036

Hartford Graduate Center
Hartford, CT 06120
(203) 548-2400

Yale University
1502A Yale Station
New Haven, CT 06520
(203) 432-1900

George Washington University
Washington, DC 20052
(202) 994-6040

Howard University
2400 6th Street N.W.
Washington, DC 20059
(202) 686-6634

Florida International University
Tamiami Trail and 107th Avenue
Miami, FL 33177
(305) 554-3421

University of Florida
Gainesville, FL 32611
(904) 392-1365

University of Miami
Box 248025
Coral Gables, FL 33124
(305) 284-4323

Georgia State University
University Plaza
Atlanta, GA 30303-3085
(404) 651-2365

Northwestern University
1801 Hinman Avenue
Evanston, IL 60201
(312) 491-7271

Rush University
1653 West Congress Parkway
Chicago, IL 60612
(312) 942-5000

University of Chicago
1116 East 59th Street
Chicago, IL 60637
(312) 702-8650

**Indiana University-Purdue University
at Indianapolis**
355 N. Lansing
Indianapolis, IN 46202
(317) 274-2306

University of Iowa
Iowa City, IA 52242
(319) 335-3847

University of Kansas
Lawrence, KS 66045
(913) 864-3911

Tulane University of Louisiana
6823 St. Charles Avenue
New Orleans, LA 70118
(504) 865-5731

Boston University
121 Bay State Road
Boston, MA 02215
(617) 353-2318

Simmons College
300 The Fenway
Boston, MA 02115
(617) 738-2107

University of Massachusetts at Amherst
University Admissions Center
Amherst, MA 01003
(413) 545-0222

University of Massachusetts Medical School
55 Lake Avenue North
Worcester, MA 01605
(508) 856-0011

University of Michigan
Ann Arbor, MI 48109
(313) 764-7433

University of Minnesota, Twin Cities Campus
231 Pillsbury Drive S.E.
240 Williamson Hall
Minneapolis, MN 55455
(612) 625-2008

University of Missouri—Columbia
Columbia, MO 65211
(314) 882-7786

St. Louis University
221 North Grand Boulevard
St. Louis, MO 63103
(314) 658-2500

Washington University
Lindell and Skinner Boulevards
St. Louis, MO 63130
(314) 889-6000

City University of New York
101 West 31st Street
Sixth floor
New York, NY 10001-3503
(212) 947-4800

Cornell University
Ithaca, NY 14850
(607) 255-5241

New York University
22 Washington Square North
New York, NY 10011
(212) 998-4533

Union College
Schenectady, NY 12308
(518) 370-6112

Duke University
2138 Campus Drive
Durham, NC 27706
(919) 684-3214

Cleveland State University
Euclid Avenue at East 24th Street
Cleveland, OH 44115
(216) 687-3755

Ohio State University
1800 Cannon Drive
Columbus, OH 43210
(614) 292-3980

Xavier University
3800 Victory Parkway
Cincinnati, OH 45207
(513) 745-3301

University of Oklahoma
660 Parrington Oval
Norman, OK 73019
(405) 325-2251

Temple University
Broad Street and Montgomery Avenue
Philadelphia, PA 19122
(215) 787-7000

University of Pennsylvania
1 College Hall
Philadelphia, PA 19104-6376
(215) 898-7507

University of Pittsburgh
Second Floor, Bruce Hall
Pittsburgh, PA 15260
(412) 624-7488

Widener University
Chester, PA 19013
(215) 499-4126

University of Puerto Rico at San Juan
GPO Box 4984-G
San Juan, PR 00936
(809) 250-0000

Medical University of South Carolina
171 Ashley Avenue
Charleston, SC 29425
(803) 792-2300

University of South Carolina
Columbia, SC 29208
(803) 777-7700

Memphis State University
Memphis, TN 38152
(901) 454-2169

Baylor University
Waco, TX 76798
(817) 755-1011

Trinity University
715 Stadium Drive
San Antonio, TX 78284
(512) 736-7207

University of Houston—Clear Lake
2700 Bay Area Boulevard
Houston, TX 77062
(713) 488-9240

University of Washington
1400 Northeast Campus Parkway
Seattle, WA 98195
(206) 543-9686

University of Wisconsin, Madison
500 Lincoln Drive
Madison, WI 53706
(608) 262-3961

DISPENSING OPTICIAN

(Programs accredited by the Commission on Opticianry Accreditation)

Pima Community College
Ophthalmic Dispensing Technology
2202 West Anklam Road
Tucson, AZ 85709
(602) 884-6916

Cañada College
Ophthalmic Dispensing
4200 Farm Hill Boulevard
Redwood City, CA 94061
(415) 306-3293

Middlesex Community College
Ophthalmic Design and Dispensing
100 Training Hill Road
Middletown, CT 06457
(203) 344-7599

Hillsborough Community College
Ophthalmic Dispensing
P.O. Box 30030
Tampa, FL 33630
(813) 253-7000

Miami-Dade Community College
Vision Care Technology/Opticianry
950 N.W. 20th Street
Miami, FL 33127
(305) 347-4032

DeKalb Technical Institute
Ophthalmic Dispensing Technology
495 North Indian Creek Drive
Clarkston, GA 30021
(404) 297-9522, ext. 207

Newbury College, Inc.
Ophthalmic Dispensing
129 Fisher Avenue
Brookline, MA 02146-5796
(617) 730-7054

Ferris State University
Opticianry
V.F.S. 424
Big Rapids, MI 49307
(616) 592-2224

Camden County College
Ophthalmic Science
P.O. Box 200
Blackwood, NJ 08012
(609) 227-7200 ext. 322

Essex County College
Ophthalmic Dispensing
303 University Avenue
Newark, NJ 07102
(201) 877-3367

Southwestern Indian Polytechnic Institute
Optical Technology-Dispensing
9169 Coors Road, N.W.
Albuquerque, NM 87184
(505) 897-5359

Erie Community College
Ophthalmic Dispensing
6205 Main Street
Williamsville, NY 14221-7095
(716) 634-0800, ext. 400

Interboro Institute
Ophthalmic Dispensing
450 West 56th Street
New York, NY 10019
(212) 399-0091

Mater Dei College
Ophthalmic Dispensing
Riverside Drive
Ogdensburg, NY 13669
(315) 393-5930

New York City Technical College
Ophthalmic Dispensing
300 Jay Street
Brooklyn, NY 11201
(718) 260-5298

Durham Technical Community College
Opticianry
1637 Lawson Street
Durham, NC 27703
(919) 598-9239

Cuyahoga Community College
Ophthalmic Dispensing Technology
2900 Community College Avenue
Cleveland, OH 44115
(216) 987-4000

Puerto Rico Tech Junior College, Inc.
Ophthalmic Dispensing
Avenida Ponce de Leon, #703
Hato Rey, PR 00917
(809) 751-0133

Roane State Community College
Opticianry
Patton Lane
Harriman, TN 37748
(615) 882-4594

El Paso Community College
Ophthalmic Technology
P.O. Box 20500
El Paso, TX 79998
(915) 594-2000

J. Sargeant Reynolds Community College
Opticianry
P.O. Box C-32040
Richmond, VA 23261-2040
(804) 786-5298

**Naval Ophthalmic Support & Training Activity/
Thomas Nelson Community College**
Ophthalmic Dispensing
Yorktown, VA 23691-5071
(804) 887-7148

Seattle Central Community College
Ophthalmic Dispensing Technology
1701 Broadway
Seattle, WA 98122
(206) 344-4321

PHARMACIST

*(All programs accredited by the American Council on Pharmaceutical Education. Those programs marked # offer only the doctor of pharmacy degree; those marked * offer both bachelor of pharmacy and doctor of pharmacy degrees; those marked with + offer only the bachelor of pharmacy.)*

* Auburn University
Samford Hall
Auburn, AL 36849-3501
(205) 844-4080

* Samford University
800 Lakeshore Drive
Birmingham, AL 35229
(205) 870-2901

 # University of Arizona
Tucson, AZ 85721
(602) 621-3237

 # University of Arkansas at Little Rock
2801 South University
Little Rock, AR 52204
(501) 569-3127

 # University of California, San Francisco
3rd Avenue and Parnassus
San Francisco, CA 94143
(415) 476-8280

 # University of the Pacific
Stockton, CA 95211
(209) 946-2211

 # University of Southern California
SAS 342-University Park
Los Angeles, CA 90089-0911
(213) 743-6741

+ University of Colorado at Boulder
Boulder, CO 80309
(303) 492-6301

+ University of Connecticut
Storrs, CT 06268
(203) 486-3137

* Howard University
2400 6th Street N.W.
Washington, DC 20059
(202) 686-6634

* Florida Agricultural and Mechanical University
Martin Luther King Jr. Boulevard
Tallahassee, FL 32307
(904) 599-3796

* Southeastern College of Osteopathic Medicine
1750 N.E. 168th Street
North Miami Beach, FL 33162
(305) 949-4000

* University of Florida
Gainesville, FL 32611
(904) 392-1365

Mercer University
1400 Coleman Avenue
Macon, GA 31207
(912) 744-2650

* University of Georgia
Athens, GA 30602
(404) 542-2112

* Idaho State University
Pocatello, ID 83209
(208) 236-3277

University of Illinois at Chicago
Box 5220
Chicago, IL 60680
(312) 996-0998

+ Butler University
46th at Sunset Avenue
Indianapolis, IN 46208
(317) 283-9255

* Purdue University
West Lafayette, IN 47907
(317) 494-1776

+ Drake University
Des Moines, IA 50311
(515) 271-3181

* University of Iowa
Iowa City, IA 52242
(319) 335-3847

* University of Kansas
Lawrence, KS 66045
(913) 864-3911

* University of Kentucky
100 W.D. Funkhouser Bldg.
Lexington, KY 40506-0054
(606) 257-2000

+ Northeast Louisiana University
700 University Avenue
Monroe, LA 71209-1110
(318) 342-4170

* Xavier University of Louisiana
7325 Palmetto Street
New Orleans, LA 70125
(504) 486-7411

* University of Maryland, Baltimore County
5401 Wilkens Avenue
Baltimore, MD 21228
(410) 455-2291

* Massachusetts College of Pharmacy and Allied Health Sciences
179 Longwood Avenue
Boston, MA 02115
(617) 732-2800

* Northeastern University
360 Huntington Avenue
Boston, MA 02115
(617) 437-2200

* Ferris State University
Big Rapids, MI 49307
(616) 592-2100

* Wayne State University
1142 Mackenzie Hall
Detroit, MI 48202
(313) 577-3577

University of Michigan
Ann Arbor, MI 48109
(313) 764-7433

* University of Minnesota, Twin Cities Campus
231 Pillsbury Drive S.E.
240 Williamson Hall
Minneapolis, MN 55455
(612) 625-2008

+ University of Mississippi
University, MS 38677
(601) 232-7226

* St. Louis College of Pharmacy
4588 Parkview Place
St. Louis, MO 63110
(314) 367-8700

* University of Missouri—Kansas City
5100 Rockhill Road
Kansas City, MO 64110
(816) 276-1111

* **University of Montana**
Missoula, MT 59812
(406) 243-6266

* **Creighton University**
2500 California Street
Omaha, NE 68178
(402) 280-2703

\# **University of Nebraska Medical Center**
42nd and Dewey Avenue
Omaha, NE 68105
(402) 554-2800

* **Rutgers University College of Pharmacy**
P.O. Box 2101
New Brunswick, NJ 08903
(908) 932-3770

\+ **University of New Mexico**
Albuquerque, NM 87131
(505) 277-2446

* **Albany College of Pharmacy of Union University**
106 New Scotland Avenue
Albany, NY 12208
(518) 445-5544

\+ **Long Island University—University Center**
Brookville, NY 11548
(516) 299-2413

* **St. John's University**
Grand Central and Utopia Parkways
Jamaica, NY 11439
(718) 990-6161

* **State University of New York at Buffalo**
1300 Elmwood Avenue
Buffalo, NY 14222
(716) 878-5511

\# **Campbell University**
P.O. Box 546
Buies Creek, NC 27506
(919) 893-4111, ext. 2275

* **University of North Carolina at Chapel Hill**
Chapel Hill, NC 27514
(919) 966-3621

\# **North Dakota State University**
University Station
Fargo, ND 58105
(701) 237-7752

\+ **Ohio Northern University**
South Main Street
Ada, OH 45810
(419) 772-2260

* **Ohio State University**
1800 Cannon Drive
Columbus, OH 43210
(614) 292-3980

* **University of Cincinnati**
Clifton Avenue
Cincinnati, OH 45221
(513) 475-3425

* **University of Toledo**
2801 W. Bancroft
Toledo, OH 43606
(419) 537-2696

\+ **Southwestern Oklahoma State University**
Weatherford, OK 73096
(405) 772-6611

* **University of Oklahoma**
660 Parrington Oval
Norman, OK 73019
(405) 325-2251

\+ **Oregon State University**
Corvallis, OR 97331
(503) 754-4411

* **Duquesne University**
600 Forbes Avenue
Pittsburgh, PA 15282
(412) 434-6220

* **Philadelphia College of Pharmacy and Science**
43rd Street at Woodland Avenue
Philadelphia, PA 19104
(215) 596-8810

\+ **Temple University**
Broad Street and Montgomery Avenue
Philadelphia, PA 19122
(215) 787-7000

+ **University of Pittsburgh**
Second Floor, Bruce Hall
Pittsburgh, PA 15260
(412) 624-7488

+ **University of Puerto Rico, San Juan**
GPO Box 4984-G
San Juan, PR 00936
(809) 250-0000

* **University of Rhode Island**
Kingston, RI 02881
(401) 792-9800

* **Medical University of South Carolina**
171 Ashley Avenue
Charleston, SC 29425
(803) 792-2300

* **University of South Carolina**
Columbia, SC 29208
(803) 777-7700

+ **University of South Dakota**
Vermillion, SD 57069
(605) 677-5434

University of Tennessee, Memphis
62 South Dunlap
Memphis, TN 38163
(901) 528-5560

* **Texas Southern University**
3100 Cleburne Avenue
Houston, TX 77004
(713) 527-7011

+ **University of Houston at University Park**
4800 Calhoun
Houston, TX 77004
(713) 749-2321

* **University of Texas at Austin**
University Station
Austin, TX 78712-1159
(512) 471-1711

* **University of Utah**
Salt Lake City, UT 84112
(801) 581-7281

* **Virginia Commonwealth University**
910 West Franklin Street
Box 2526
Richmond, VA 23284
(804) 257-6124

+ **Washington State University**
342 French Administration
Pullman, WA 99164
(509) 335-5586

* **University of Washington**
1400 Northeast Campus Parkway
Seattle, WA 98195
(206) 543-9686

* **West Virginia University**
Morgantown, WV 26506
(304) 293-2121

* **University of Wisconsin, Madison**
500 Lincoln Drive
Madison, WI 53706
(608) 262-3961

+ **University of Wyoming**
Box 3435
Laramie, WY 82071
(307) 766-5160

RADIOLOGIC TECHNOLOGIST

A total of 661 hospital, college, and university-based programs throughout the United States and Puerto Rico offer fully accredited training for Radiologic Technologists, often called Radiographers. These programs are accredited by the Division of Allied Health Education and Accreditation of the American Medical Association. There are an additional 104 accredited programs for Radiation Therapy Technologists. Radiation Therapy Technologists are more highly educated and trained, take responsibility for actually administering radiation therapy, and accordingly are more highly paid.

PHYSICAL THERAPIST

*(All programs accredited by the American Physical Therapy Association. Programs marked * offer an approved Master's program as well as the under-graduate degree.)*

* University of Alabama at Birmingham
University Station
Birmingham, AL 35294
(205) 934-8221

University of South Alabama
307 University Boulevard
Mobile, AL 36688
(205) 460-6141

* Northern Arizona University
Box 4082
Flagstaff, AZ 86011
(602) 523-5511

* University of Central Arkansas
Conway, AR 72032
(501) 450-3128

California State University, Fresno
Shaw and Cedar Avenues
Fresno, CA 93740
(209) 294-2191

California State University, Long Beach
1250 Bellflower Boulevard
Long Beach, CA 90840
(213) 498-4111

California State University, Northridge
18111 Nordhoff Street
Northridge, CA 91330
(213) 885-1200

* Loma Linda University
Loma Linda, CA 92350
(714) 785-2118

Mount St. Mary's College
12001 Chalon Road
Los Angeles, CA 90049
(213) 476-2237

* University of the Pacific
Stockton, CA 95211
(209) 946-2211

* University of Southern California
SAS 342-University Park
Los Angeles, CA 90089-0911
(213) 743-6741

University of Colorado at Denver
1200 Larimer Street
Denver, CO 80204-5300
(303) 556-2275

Quinnipiac College
Mount Carmel Avenue
Hamden, CT 06518
(203) 288-5251, ext. 338

University of Connecticut
Storrs, CT 06268
(203) 486-3137

University of Delaware
Newark, DE 19716
(302) 451-8123

Howard University
2400 6th Street N.W.
Washington, DC 20059
(202) 686-6634

Florida Agricultural and Mechanical University
Martin Luther King Jr. Boulevard
Tallahassee, FL 32307
(904) 599-3796

Florida International University
Tamiami Trail and 107th Avenue
Miami, FL 33177
(305) 554-3421

University of Florida
Gainesville, FL 32611
(904) 392-1365

* University of Miami
Box 248025
Coral Gables, FL 33124
(305) 284-4323

* Emory University
Atlanta, GA 30322
(404) 727-6036

Georgia State University
University Plaza
Atlanta, GA 30303-3085
(404) 651-2365

Medical College of Georgia
1120 15th Street
Augusta, GA 30912
(404) 721-2725

Northern Illinois University
5500 North St. Louis Avenue
Chicago, IL 60625
(312) 794-2600

Northwestern University
1801 Hinman Avenue
Evanston, IL 60201
(312) 491-7271

University of Health Sciences/Chicago Medical School
3333 Green Bay Road
Chicago, IL 60604
(708) 578-3000

University of Illinois at Chicago
Box 5220
Chicago, IL 60680
(312) 996-0998

Indiana University-Purdue University at Indianapolis
355 North Lansing
Indianapolis, IN 46202
(317) 274-2306

University of Evansville
1800 Lincoln Avenue
Evansville, IN 47722
(812) 479-2468

* University of Indianapolis
1400 E. Hanna Avenue
Indianapolis, IN 46227
(317) 788-3216

* University of Iowa
Iowa City, IA 52242
(319) 335-3847

* University of Kansas
Lawrence, KS 66045
(913) 864-3911

Wichita State University
1845 Fairmount
Wichita, KS 67208
(316) 689-3085

University of Kentucky
100 W.D. Funkhouser Bldg.
Lexington, KY 40506-0054
(606) 257-2000

Louisiana State University Medical Center
1440 Canal Street
Suite 1510
New Orleans, LA 70112

University of Maryland, Baltimore County
5401 Wilkens Avenue
Baltimore, MD 21228
(410) 455-2291

University of Maryland, Eastern Shore
Princess Anne, MD 21853
(410) 651-2200

* Boston University
121 Bay State Road
Boston, MA 02215
(617) 353-2318

Northeastern University
360 Huntington Avenue
Boston, MA 02115
(617) 437-2200

* Simmons College
300 The Fenway
Boston, MA 02115
(617) 738-2107

* Springfield College
Springfield, MA 01109
(413) 788-3136

* University of Lowell
One University Avenue
Lowell, MA 01854
(508) 452-5000, ext. 2413

* Andrews University
Berrien Springs, MI 49104
(616) 471-3303

* Grand Valley State University
College Landing
Allendale, MI 49401
(616) 895-2025

* Oakland University
Wilson Hall-205
Rochester, MI 48039-4401
(313) 377-3360

* University of Michigan, Flint
Flint, MI 48502-2186
(313) 762-3300

Wayne State University
1142 Mackenzie Hall
Detroit, MI 48202
(313) 577-3577

* College of Saint Scholastica
1200 Kenwood Avenue
Duluth, MN 55811
(218) 723-6046

Mayo Foundation
200 First Street S.W.
Rochester, MN 55905
(507) 284-3671

University of Minnesota, Twin Cities Campus
231 Pillsbury Drive, S.E.
240 Williamson Hall
Minneapolis, MN 55455
(612) 625-2008

University of Mississippi, School of Medicine
2500 North State Street
Jackson, MS 39216
(601) 984-1010

Rockhurst College
1100 Rockhurst Road
Kansas City, MO 64110
(816) 926-4100

St. Louis University
221 North Grand Boulevard
St. Louis, MO 63103
(314) 658-2500

University of Missouri, Columbia
Columbia, MO 65211
(314) 882-7786

University of Montana
Missoula, MT 59812
(406) 243-6266

* University of Nebraska Medical Center
42nd and Dewey Avenue
Omaha, NE 68105
(402) 559-4204

Kean College of New Jersey
Morris Avenue
Union, NJ 07083
(201) 527-2195

* Rutgers University
New Brunswick, NJ 08903
(201) 932-1766

Stockton State College
Jim Leeds Road
Pomona, NJ 08240
(609) 652-4261

University of New Mexico
Albuquerque, NM 87131
(505) 277-2446

Columbia College/Columbia University
212 Hamilton Hall
New York, NY 10027
(212) 854-2521

Daemen College
4380 Main Street
Amherst, NY 14226
(716) 839-1820

Hunter College (CUNY)
695 Park Avenue
New York, NY 10021
(212) 772-4490

* Ithaca College
Danby Road
Ithaca, NY 14850
(607) 274-3124

* Long Island University—University Center
Brookville, NY 11548
(516) 299-2413

New York University
22 Washington Square North
New York, NY 10011
(212) 998-4533

Russel Sage College
45 Ferry Street
Troy, NY 12180
(518) 270-2217

State University of New York at Buffalo
1300 Elmwood Avenue
Buffalo, NY 14222
(716) 878-5511

State University of New York, Health Science
Center—Brooklyn
450 Clarkson Avenue
Brooklyn, NY 11203
(718) 270-1000

State University of New York, Health Science
Center—Syracuse
155 Elizabeth Blackwell Street
Syracuse, NY 13210
(315) 473-4570

State University of New York at Stony Brook
Stony Brook, NY 11794
(516) 632-6868

* Touro College
844 Avenue of the Americas
New York, NY 10001-4104
(212) 447-0700

Duke University
2138 Campus Drive
Durham, NC 27706
(919) 684-3214

East Carolina University
East Fifth Street
Greenville, NC 27858-4353
(919) 757-6640

University of North Carolina at Chapel Hill
Chapel Hill, NC 27514
(919) 966-3621

University of North Dakota
Box 8095, University Station
Grand Forks, ND 58202
(701) 777-2711

Cleveland State University
Euclid Avenue at East 24th Street
Cleveland, OH 44115
(216) 687-3755

Medical College of Ohio at Toledo
Caller Service No. 10008
Toledo, OH 43699
(419) 381-4107

Ohio State University
1800 Cannon Drive
Columbus, OH 43210
(614) 292-3980

Ohio University
Athens, OH 45701
(614) 593-4100

Langston University
P.O. Box 838
Langston, OK 73050
(405) 466-2231

University of Oklahoma Medical Center
P.O. Box 2690
Oklahoma City, OK 73190
(405) 271-2265

* Pacific University
Forest Grove, OR 97116
(503) 359-2218

* Beaver College
Easton and Church Roads
Glenside, PA 19038
(215) 572-2910

* Hahnemann University, School of Health Sciences
201 North 15th Street
Mail Stop 506
Philadelphia, PA 19102-1192
(215) 448-8288

* Philadelphia College of Pharmacy and Science
43rd at Woodland Avenue
Philadelphia, PA 19104
(215) 596-8810

* Temple University
Broad Street and Montgomery Avenue
Philadelphia, PA 19122
(215) 787-7000

* Thomas Jefferson University/College of Allied
Health Sciences
1020 Locust Street
Philadelphia, PA 19107
(215) 929-8890

* University of Pittsburgh
Second Floor, Bruce Hall
Pittsburgh, PA 15260
(412) 624-7488

University of Scranton
Scranton, PA 18510-2192
(717) 961-7540

University of Puerto Rico
GPO Box 4984-G
San Juan, PR 00936
(809) 250-0000

Medical University of South Carolina
171 Ashley Avenue
Charleston, SC 29425
(803) 792-2300

Maryville College
Maryville, TN 37801
(615) 982-6412

University of Tennessee, Memphis
62 South Dunlap
Memphis, TN 38163
(901) 528-5560

Southwest Texas State University
San Marcos, TX 78666
(512) 245-2364

Texas Tech University
P.O. Box 40409
Lubbock, TX 79409
(806) 742-3652

* Texas Woman's University
P.O. Box 22909 T.W.U. Station
Denton, TX 76204
(817) 893-3000

University of Texas Health Science Center
at San Antonio
7703 Floyd Curl Drive
San Antonio, TX 78284
(512) 567-7000

University of Texas Medical Branch
541 Administration Building
300 University Boulevard
Galveston, TX 77550
(409) 761-1011

University of Texas Southwestern Medical Center
at Dallas
5323 Henry Hines Boulevard
Dallas, TX 75235
(214) 688-3111

University of Utah
Salt Lake City, UT 84112
(801) 581-7281

University of Vermont
194 South Prospect Street
Burlington, VT 05401-3596
(802) 656-3370

Old Dominion University
Norfolk, VA 23529-0050
(804) 683-3637

Virginia Commonwealth University
910 West Franklin Street
Box 2526
Richmond, VA 23284
(804) 257-6124

Eastern Washington University
M.S. 148 Admissions Office
Cheney, WA 99004
(509) 359-2397

* University of Puget Sound
1500 North Warner Street
Tacoma, WA 98416
(206) 756-3211

University of Washington
1400 Northeast Campus Parkway
Seattle, WA 98195
(206) 543-9686

West Virginia University
Morgantown, WV 26506
(304) 293-2121

Marquette University
615 North 11th Street
Milwaukee, WI 53233
(414) 288-7302

University of Wisconsin—LaCrosse
1725 State Street
LaCrosse, WI 54601
(608) 785-8067

University of Wisconsin—Madison
500 Lincoln Drive
Madison, WI 53706
(608) 262-3961

PHYSICAL THERAPY ASSISTANT

(All programs accredited by the American Physical Therapy Association)

University of Alabama at Birmingham
University Station
Birmingham, AL 35294
(205) 934-8221

University of Central Arkansas
Conway, AR 73032
(501) 450-3128

Cerritos College
11110 East Alondra Boulevard
Norwalk, CA 90650
(213) 860-2451

DeAnza College
21250 Stevens Creek Boulevard
Cupertino, CA 95014
(408) 864-5678

Loma Linda University
Loma Linda, CA 92350
(714) 785-2118

Mount St. Mary's College
12001 Chalon Road
Los Angeles, CA 90049
(213) 476-2237

San Diego Mesa College
7250 Mesa College Drive
San Diego, CA 92111
(619) 560-2600

Housatonic Community College
510 Barnum Avenue
Bridgeport, CT 06608
(203) 579-6400

Delaware Technical and Community College Wilmington Campus
333 Shipley Street
Wilmington, DE 19801
(302) 571-5300

Broward Community College
225 East Las Olas Boulevard
Fort Lauderdale, FL 33301
(305) 475-6500

Miami-Dade Community College
300 N.E. Second Avenue
Miami, FL 33132
(305) 347-1000

Pensacola Junior College
1000 College Boulevard
Pensacola, FL 32504
(904) 484-1000

St. Petersburg Junior College
8580 66th Street North
Pinellas Park, FL 34665-1207
(813) 341-3600

Gwinnett Area Technical School
1250 Atkinson Road
Box 1505
Lawrenceville, GA 30246
(404) 962-7580

Kapiolani Community College
4303 Diamond Head Road
Honolulu, HI 96816
(808) 734-9111

Belleville Area College
2500 Carlyle Road
Belleville, IL 62221
(618) 235-2700

Illinois Central College
East Peoria, IL 61635
(309) 693-5011

Morton College
3801 South Central Avenue
Cicero, IL 60650
(708) 656-8000

Oakton Community College
1600 East Golf Road
Des Plaines, IL 60016
(708) 635-1600

Southern Illinois University at Carbondale
Carbondale, IL 62901
(618) 453-4381

University of Evansville
1800 Lincoln Avenue
Evansville, IN 47722
(812) 479-2468

Vincennes University
1002 North First Street
Vincennes, IN 47591
(812) 885-4313

Colby Community College
1255 South Range
Colby, KS 67701
(913) 462-3984

Washburn University
1700 College
Topeka, KS 66621
(913) 295-6625

Jefferson Community College
109 East Broadway
Louisville, KY 40202
(502) 584-0181

Paducah Community College
P.O. Box 7380
Paducah, KY 42002
(502) 554-9200

Somerset Community College
808 Monticello Road
Somerset, KY 42501
(606) 679-8501

Community College of Baltimore, Liberty Campus
2901 Liberty Heights Avenue
Baltimore, MD 21215
(410) 396-0203

Becker Junior College
61 Sever Street
Worcester, MA 01609
(508) 791-9241

Lasell College
1844 Commonwealth Avenue
Newton, MA 02166
(617) 243-2225

Newbury College
129 Fisher Avenue
Brookline, MA 02146
(617) 730-7007

North Shore Community College
3 Essex Street
Beverly, MA 01915
(508) 922-6722

Springfield Technical Community College
Springfield, MA 01105
(413) 781-7822

Delta College
University Center, MI 48710
(517) 686-9092

Kellogg Community College
450 North Avenue
Battle Creek, MI 49016
(616) 965-3931

Macomb Community College
14500 Twelve Mile Road
Warren, MI 48093
(313) 445-7000

Anoka Area Voc Tech Institute
1355 West Main Street
Box 191
Anoka, MN 55303
(612) 427-1880

College of Saint Catherine
2004 Randolph Street
St. Paul, MN 55105
(612) 690-6505

Penn Valley Community College
3201 Southwest Trafficway
Kansas City, MO 64111
(816) 932-7600

St. Louis Community College at Meramec
11333 Big Bend
Kirkwood, MO 63122
(314) 966-7500

New Hampshire Vocational-Technical College
Berlin, NH 03570
(603) 752-1113

Atlantic Community College
Black Horse Pike
Mays Landing, NJ 08330
(609) 625-1111

Essex County College
303 University Avenue
Newark, NJ 07102
(201) 877-3000

Fairleigh Dickinson University
West Passaic and Montross Avenues
Rutherford, NJ 07070
(201) 460-5267

Union County College
1033 Springfield Avenue
Cranford, NJ 07016
(908) 709-7000

Broome Community College
Upper Front Street, Box 1017
Binghamton, NY 13902
(607) 771-5000

LaGuardia Community College (CUNY)
31-10 Thomson Avenue
Long Island City, NY 11101
(718) 482-5000

Maria College
700 New Scotland Avenue
Albany, NY 12208
(518) 438-3111

Nassau Community College
Stewart Avenue
Garden City, NY 11530
(516) 222-7355

Onondaga Community College
Route 173
Syracuse, NY 13215
(315) 469-7741

Suffolk County Community College, Eastern Campus
Speonk-Riverhead Road
Riverhead, NY 11901
(516) 548-2500

Central Piedmont Community College
Box 35009
Charlotte, NC 28235
(704) 342-6633

Fayetteville Technical Community College
P.O. Box 35236
Fayetteville, NC 28303
(919) 323-1961

Martin Community College
Kehukee Park Road
Williamston, NC 27892
(919) 792-1521

Nash Community College
Old Carriage Road
Rocky Mount, NC 27804
(919) 443-4011

Central Ohio Technical College
University Drive
Newark, OH 43055
(614) 366-1351

Cuyahoga Community College
700 Carnegie Avenue
Cleveland, OH 44115
(216) 987-4000

Kent State University
Kent, OH 44242
(216) 672-2444

Shawnee State University
940 Second Street
Portsmouth, OH 45662
(614) 354-3205

Sinclair Community College
444 West Third Street
Dayton, OH 45402
(513) 226-2500

Stark Technical College
6200 Frank Avenue N.W.
Canton, OH 44720
(216) 494-6170

University of Cincinnati
Clifton Avenue
Cincinnati, OH 45221
(513) 475-3425

Oklahoma City Community College
7777 South May
Oklahoma City, OK 73159
(405) 682-1611

Tulsa Junior College
6111 East Shelly Drive 200
Tulsa, OK 74135
(918) 587-6561

Mount Hood Community College
Gresham, OR 97030
(503) 667-6422

Alvernia College
Reading, PA 19607
(215) 775-0525

Central Pennsylvania Business School
College Hill
Summerdale, PA 17093-0309
(717) 732-0702

Community College of Allegheny County
808 Ridge Avenue
Pittsburgh, PA 15212
(412) 237-2525

Hahnemann University/School of Health Sciences
201 N. 15th Street
Mail Stop 506
Philadelphia, PA 19102-1192
(215) 448-8288

Harcum Junior College
Bryn Mawr, PA 19010
(215) 526-6050

Lehigh County Community College
2370 Main Street
Schnecksville, PA 18078
(215) 799-2121

Pennsylvania State University—Hazelton Campus
Highacres
Hazelton, PA 18201
(717) 450-3000

Pennsylvania State University—Mont Alto Campus
Mont Alto, PA 17237
(717) 749-3111

University of Puerto Rico, Humacao University College
CUH Station
Humacao, PR 00661
(809) 850-0000

University of Puerto Rico, Ponce Technological University College
Box 7186
Ponce, PR 00732
(809) 844-8181

Greenville Technical College
P.O. Box 5616, Station B
Greenville, SC 29606
(803) 250-8000

Trident Technical College
P.O. Box 1037
Charleston, SC 29411
(803) 572-6111

Chattanooga State Technical Community College
4501 Amnicola Highway
Chattanooga, TN 37406
(615) 697-4400

Roane State Community College
Patton Lane
Harriman, TN 37748
(615) 354-3000

Shelby State Community College
Box 40568
Memphis, TN 38174-0568
(901) 528-6700

Volunteer State Community College
Nashville Pike
Gallatin, TN 37066
(615) 452-8600

Walters State Community College
500 South Davy Crockett Parkway
Morristown, TN 37813
(615) 587-9722

Amarillo College
Box 447
Amarillo, TX 79178
(806) 371-5000

Austin Community College
P.O. Box 2285
Austin, TX 78768
(512) 483-7000

Houston Community College
22 Waugh Drive
Houston, TX 77007
(713) 869-5021

Kilgore College
1100 Broadway
Kilgore, TX 75662
(214) 984-8531

Laredo Junior College
West End Washington Street
Laredo, TX 78040
(512) 722-0521

McClennan Community College
1400 College Drive
Waco, TX 76708
(817) 756-6551

Pan American University
1201 W. University Drive
Edinburg, TX 78539
(512) 381-2011

St. Philip's College
211 Nevada
San Antonio, TX 78203
(512) 531-3200

Tarrant County Junior College
1500 Houston Street
Fort Worth, TX 76102-6599
(817) 336-7851

Community Hospital College of Health Sciences
Box 1951
Roanoke, VA 24008
(703) 985-8483

Northern Virginia Community College
8333 Little River Turnpike
Annandale, VA 22003-3796
(703) 323-3000

Tidewater Community College
State Route 135
Portsmouth, VA 23703
(804) 484-2121

Wytheville Community College
1000 East Main Street
Wytheville, VA 24382
(703) 228-5541

Green River Community College
Auburn, WA 98002
(206) 833-9111

Blackhawk Technical College
P.O. Box 5009
6004 Prairie Road
Janesville, WI 53545
(608) 756-4121

Milwaukee Area Technical College
700 West State Street
Milwaukee, WI 53233
(414) 278-6600

Northeast Wisconsin Technical College
2740 West Mason Street
Green Bay, WI 54307
(414) 498-5400

MUSIC THERAPIST

(All programs approved by the National Association for Music Therapy, Inc.)

University of Alabama
Box UA
Tuscaloosa, AL 45387
(205) 348-5666

Arizona State University
Tempe, AZ 85287
(602) 965-7788

California State University, Long Beach
1250 Bellflower Boulevard
Long Beach, CA 90840
(213) 498-4111

California State University, Northridge
18111 Nordhoff Street
Northridge, CA 91330
(213) 885-1200

University of the Pacific
Stockton, CA 95211
(209) 946-2211

Colorado State University
Fort Collins, CO 80523
(303) 491-7008

Howard University
2400 Sixth Street N.W.
Washington, DC 20059
(202) 686-6634

Florida State University
Tallahassee, FL 32306-1009
(904) 644-6200

University of Miami
Box 248025
Coral Gables, FL 33124
(305) 284-4323

Georgia College
231 West Hancock Street Campus
P.O. Box 023
Milledgeville, GA 31061
(912) 453-5234

University of Georgia
Athens, GA 30602
(404) 542-2112

Illinois State University
Normal, IL 61761
(309) 438-2181

Western Illinois University
900 West Adams Street
Macomb, IL 61455
(309) 298-1891

Indiana University—Purdue University at Fort Wayne
2101 Coliseum Boulevard
Fort Wayne, IN 46805-1499
(219) 481-6812

University of Evansville
1800 Lincoln Avenue
Evansville, IN 47722
(812) 479-2237

University of Iowa
Iowa City, IA 52242
(319) 335-3847

Wartburg College
Waverly, IA 50677
(319) 352-8264

University of Kansas
Lawrence, KS 66045
(913) 864-3911

Loyola University
6363 St. Charles Avenue
New Orleans, LA 70118
(504) 865-3240

Anna Maria College
Sunset Lane
Paxton, MA 01612
(508) 757-4586

Eastern Michigan University
Ypsilanti, MI 48197
(313) 487-3060

Michigan State University
East Lansing, MI 48824
(517) 355-8332

Wayne State University
1142 Mackenzie Hall
Detroit, MI 48202
(313) 577-3577

Western Michigan University
Kalamazoo, MI 49008
(616) 383-1950

Augsburg College
731 21st Avenue South
Minneapolis, MN 55454
(612) 330-1001

University of Minnesota, Twin Cities Campus
231 Pillsbury Drive Southeast
240 Williamson Hall
Minneapolis, MN 55455
(612) 625-2008

William Carey College
Tuscan Avenue
Hattiesburg, MS 39401
(601) 582-5051, ext. 210

Maryville College
13550 Conway Road
St. Louis, MO 63141
(314) 576-9350

University of Missouri, Kansas City
5100 Rockhill Road
Kansas City, MO 64110
(816) 276-1111

Eastern Montana College
Billings, MT 59101
(406) 657-2158

Montclair State College
Valley Road and Norman Avenue
Upper Montclair, NJ 07043
(201) 893-4444

Eastern New Mexico University
Portales, NM 88130
(505) 562-2178

Nazareth College of Rochester
4245 East Avenue
Rochester, NY 14610
(716) 586-2525

State University of New York College at Fredonia
Fredonia, NY 14063
(716) 673-3251

State University of New York College at New Paltz
New Paltz, NY 12561
(914) 257-3200

East Carolina University
East Fifth Street
Greenville, NC 27858-4353
(919) 757-6640

Mars Hill College
Mars Hill, NC 28754
(704) 689-1201

Queens College
1900 Selwyn Avenue
Charlotte, NC 28274
(704) 337-2355

Baldwin-Wallace College
275 Eastland Road
Berea, OH 44017
(216) 826-2222

College of Mount St. Joseph
5701 Delhi Road
Mount St. Joseph, OH 45051
(513) 244-4531

Ohio University
Athens, OH 45701
(614) 593-4100

University of Dayton
300 College Park Avenue
Dayton, OH 45469
(513) 229-4411

Phillips University
Box 2000 University Station
Enid, OK 73702
(405) 237-4433

Southwestern Oklahoma State University
Weatherford, OK 73096
(405) 772-6611

Willamette University
Salem, OR 97301
(503) 730-6303

Duquesne University
600 Forbes Avenue
Pittsburgh, PA 15282
(412) 434-6220

Elizabethtown College
Elizabethtown, PA 17022
(717) 367-1151, ext. 191

Hahnemann University/School of Health Sciences
201 North 15th Street
Mail Stop 506
Philadelphia, PA 19102-1192
(215) 448-8288

Mansfield University of Pennsylvania
Academy Street
Mansfield, PA 16933
(717) 662-4243

Marywood College
2300 Adams Avenue
Scranton, PA 18509
(717) 348-6234

Slippery Rock University of Pennsylvania
Slippery Rock, PA 16057
(412) 794-7203

Temple University
Broad Street and Montgomery Avenue
Philadelphia, PA 19122
(215) 787-7000

Baptist College at Charleston
Box 10087
Charleston, SC 29411
(803) 797-4326

Tennessee Technological University
Box 5006
Cookeville, TN 38505
(615) 372-3888

Sam Houston State University
P.O. Box 2026
Huntsville, TX 77341
(409) 294-1056

Southern Methodist University
P.O. Box 296
Dallas, TX 75275
(214) 692-2058

Texas Woman's University
P.O. Box 22909 T.W.U. Station
Denton, TX 76204
(817) 898-3000

West Texas State University
Box 999
Canyon, TX 79016
(806) 656-3331

Utah State University
Logan, UT 84322
(801) 750-1006

Radford University
Radford, Va 24142
(703) 831-5371

Alverno College
3401 South 39 Street
Milwaukee, WI 53215
(414) 382-6100

University of Wisconsin—Eau Claire
Eau Claire, WI 54701
(715) 836-5415

University of Wisconsin—Milwaukee
P.O. Box 749
Milwaukee, WI 53201
(414) 229-3800

University of Wisconsin—Oshkosh
800 Algoma Boulevard
Oshkosh, WI 54901
(414) 424-0202

DANCE THERAPIST

(Graduate programs according to the American Dance Therapy Association, Inc. Schools marked * offer approved American Dance Therapy Association graduate degree programs. Those schools marked # offer undergraduate programs as well as graduate programs.)

*University of California at Los Angeles
405 Hilgard Avenue
Los Angeles, CA 90024
(213) 825-3101

California State University, Hayward
Hayward, CA 94542
(415) 881-3817

#*Naropa Institute
2130 Arapahoe Avenue
Boulder, CO 80302
(303) 444-0202, ext. 511

#Barat College
700 East Westleigh Road
Lake Forest, IL 60045
(312) 234-3000

Columbia College
600 South Michigan Avenue
Chicago, IL 60605
(312) 663-1600

#*Goucher College
Dulaney Valley Road
Baltimore, MD 21204
(410) 337-6100

Lesley College
39 Everett Street
Cambridge, MA 02138-2790
(617) 868-9600, ext. 176

*Antioch/New England Graduate School
Roxbury Street
Keene, NH 03431
(603) 357-3122

*Hunter College (City University of New York)
695 Park Avenue
New York, NY 10021
(212) 772-4490

#*New York University
22 Washington Square North
New York, NY 10011
(212) 998-4500

*Hahnemann University/School of Health Sciences
201 North 15th Street
Mail Stop 506
Philadelphia, PA 19102-1192
(215) 448-8288

#University of Wisconsin, Madison
500 Lincoln Drive
Madison, WI 53706
(608) 262-3961

VETERINARY TECHNICIAN

(Associate degree programs in animal technology accredited by the American Veterinary Medical Association. Programs marked * offer bachelor's degree programs as well. Programs marked # offer a certificate program.)

Snead State Junior College
P.O. Drawer D
Boaz, AL 35957
(205) 593-5120

Cosumnes River College
8401 Center Parkway
Sacramento, CA 95823
(916) 688-7410

Foothill College
12345 El Monte Road
Los Altos Hills, CA 94022
(415) 949-7777

Hartnell College
156 Homestead Avenue
Salinas, CA 93901
(408) 755-6700

Los Angeles Pierce College
6201 Winnetka Avenue
Woodland Hills, CA 91371
(818) 347-0551

Mt. San Antonio College
1499 North Grand Avenue
Walnut, CA 91789
(714) 594-5611

San Diego Mesa College
7250 Mesa College Drive
San Diego, CA 92111
(619) 560-2600

Yuba College
2088 North Beale Road
Marysville, CA 95901
(916) 741-6700

Colorado Mountain College, Spring Valley Campus
3000 County Road 114
Glenwood Springs, CO 81601
(303) 945-7481

*Quinnipiac College
Mount Carmel Avenue
Hamden, CT 06518
(203) 288-5251, ext. 338

St. Petersburg Junior College
8580 66th Street North
Pinellas Park, FL 34665-1207
(813) 341-3600

Fort Valley State College
805 State College Drive
Fort Valley, GA 31030
(912) 825-6211

Parkland College
2400 West Bradley Avenue
Champaign, IL 61821
(217) 351-2200

Purdue University
West Lafayette, IN 47907
(317) 494-1776

Colby Community College
1255 South Range
Colby, KS 67701
(913) 462-3984

Morehead State University
Morehead, KY 40351
(606) 783-2008

*Murray State University
15th and Main Streets
Murray, KY 42071
(507) 762-3380

Northwestern State University of Louisiana
College Avenue
Natchitoches, LA 71497
(318) 357-4503

University of Maine at Orono
Orono, ME 04469
(207) 581-1561

Essex Community College
7201 Rossville Blvd.
Baltimore County, MD 21237
(410) 682-6000

Becker Junior College
61 Sever Street
Worcester, MA 01609
(508) 791-9241

Holyoke Community College
303 Homestead Avenue
Holyoke, MA 01040
(413) 538-7000

*Mount Ida College
777 Dedham Street
Newton Centre, MA 02159
(617) 969-7000

Macomb Community College
14500 Twelve Mile Road
Warren, MI 48093
(313) 445-7000

#Michigan State University
East Lansing, MI 48824
(517) 355-8332

Wayne County Community College
801 West Fort Street
Detroit, MI 48226
(313) 496-2500

University of Minnesota—Technical College, Waseca
Waseca, MN 56093
(507) 835-1000

Hinds Community College
Raymond, MS 39154
(601) 857-5261

Jefferson College
P.O. Box 1000
Hillsboro, MO 63050
(314) 789-3951

Maple Woods Community College
2601 NE Barry Road
Kansas City, MO 64111
(816) 436-6500

Omaha College of Health Careers
1052 Park Avenue
Omaha, NE 68105
(402) 342-1818

University of Nebraska School of Technical Agriculture
Curtis, NE 69025
(308) 367-4124

Camden County College
P.O. Box 200
Blackwood, NJ 08012
(609) 227-7200

La Guardia Community College (City College of New York)
3110 Thomson Avenue
Long Island City, NY 11101
(718) 626-2700

*Mercy College
555 Broadway
Dobbs Ferry, NY 10522
(914) 693-7600

State University of New York College of Agriculture and Technology at Farmingdale
Melville Road
Farmingdale, NY 11735
(516) 420-2200

State University of New York College of Technology at Canton
Cornell Drive
Canton, NY 13617
(315) 386-7123

State University of New York College of Technology at Delhi
Delhi, NY 13753
(607) 746-4246

Central Carolina Community College
1105 Kelly Drive
Sanford, NC 27330
(919) 775-5401

*North Dakota State University
University Station
Fargo, ND 58105
(701) 237-7752

Columbus State Community College
P.O. Box 1609
Columbus, OH 43216
(614) 227-2400

University of Cincinnati, Raymond Walters College
9555 Plainfield Road
Cincinnati, OH 45236
(513) 745-5600

Murray State College
104 East 24th Street
Tishomingo, OK 73460
(405) 371-2371, ext. 171

Portland Community College
12000 Southwest 49th Avenue
Portland, OR 97207
(503) 464-3511

Harcum Junior College
Bryn Mawr, PA 19010
(215) 526-6050

Wilson College
1015 Philadelphia Avenue
Chambersburg, PA 17201
(717) 264-4141, ext. 223

Tri-County Technical College
P.O. Box 587
Pendleton, SC 29670
(803) 646-8361

National College
321 Kansas City Street
Rapid City, SD 57701
(605) 394-4824

Columbia State Community College
Box 1315
Columbia, TN 38402
(615) 388-0120

Lincoln Memorial University
Harrogate, TN 37752-0901
(615) 869-3611

Amarillo College
Box 447
Amarillo, TX 79178
(806) 371-5000

Cedar Valley College
3030 North Dallas Avenue
Lancaster, TX 75134
(214) 372-8200

North Harris County College
233 Denmar Drive, Suite 150
Houston, TX 77073
(713) 443-5400

Sul Ross State University
Alpine, TX 79832
(915) 837-8052

Texas State Technical Institute—Waco
3801 Campus Drive
Waco, TX 76705
(817) 799-3611

*Brigham Young University
Provo, UT 84602
(801) 378-2507

Blue Ridge Community College
Box 80
Weyers Cave, VA 24486
(703) 234-9261

Northern Virginia Community College
8333 Little River Turnpike
Annandale, VA 22003
(703) 323-3000

Pierce College
9401 Farwest Drive SW
Tacoma, WA 98498
(206) 964-6500

Fairmont State College
Fairmont, WV 26554
(304) 367-4141

Madison Area Technical College
3550 Anderson Street
Madison, WI 53704
(608) 246-6100

Eastern Wyoming College
3200 West C Street
Torrington, WY 82240
(307) 532-7111

GERIATRIC SOCIAL WORKER and GERIATRIC ASSESSMENT COORDINATOR

The Association for Gerontology in Higher Education has approved degree granting programs in Gerontology and Geriatrics in over 300 colleges and universities throughout the United States and in Puerto Rico and Guam. In addition, one might prepare for one of these careers by earning a degree in social work with emphasis on geriatric practice.

NURSING HOME ACTIVITIES DIRECTOR

At the present time there is no prescribed course of study leading to a career as Nursing Home Activities

Director, nor is there an established certification procedure. Courses in social work, recreation therapy, geriatrics, occupational therapy, therapeutic recreation, or rehabilitation therapy may all serve as useful bases for entry into this field. The National Association of Activity Professionals is developing jointly with the National Certification Council for Activity Professionals a five-hour "Basic Activities Director's Course." This course is offered at the association's annual convention. Other courses offered are an "Advanced Activities Director's Course" and a third-level course entitled "Activity Consultant."

RECREATIONAL THERAPIST

(Programs in Therapeutic Recreation accredited by the National Recreation and Park Association.)

California Polytechnic State University, San Luis Obispo
San Luis Obispo, CA 93407
(805) 756-2311

California State University, Chico
1st and Normal Streets
Chico, CA 95929
(916) 898-6116

California State University, Fresno
Shaw and Cedar Avenues
Fresno, CA 93740
(209) 294-2191

California State University, Northridge
18111 Nordhoff Street
Northridge, CA 91330
(213) 885-1200

California State University, Sacramento
6000 J Street
Sacramento, CA 95819
(916) 454-6011

San Diego State University
5402 College Avenue
San Diego, CA 92182-0771
(619) 594-5384

San Jose State University
Washington Square
San Jose, CA 95192-0009
(408) 924-2000

Metropolitan State College
1006 11th Street
Denver, CO 80204
(303) 556-3058

University of Northern Colorado
Greeley, CO 80639
(303) 351-2881

Gallaudet University
800 Florida Avenue N.E.
Washington, DC 20002
(202) 651-5114

Florida State University
Tallahassee, FL 32306-1009
(904) 644-6200

University of Florida
Gainesville, FL 32611
(904) 392-1365

Georgia Southern College
Box 8033
Statesboro, GA 30460
(912) 681-531

University of Georgia
Athens, GA 30602
(404) 542-2112

Aurora University
Aurora, IL 60506
(312) 844-5143

Eastern Illinois University
Charleston, IL 61920
(217) 581-2223

Illinois State University
Normal, IL 61761
(309) 438-2181

Southern Illinois University
Carbondale, IL 62901
(616) 453-4381

University of Illinois at Urbana-Champaign
506 S. Wright Street
Urbana, IL 61801
(217) 333-2033

Indiana State University
217 N. 6th Street
Terre Haute, IN 47809
(812) 237-2121

University of Indiana at Bloomington
Bloomington, IN 47405
(812) 855-0661

University of Iowa
Iowa City, IA 52242
(319) 335-3847

University of Northern Iowa
172 Gilchrist Hall
Cedar Falls, IA 50614
(319) 273-2281

Eastern Kentucky University
Lancaster Avenue
Richmond, KY 40475
(606) 622-2106

University of Kentucky
100 W.D. Funkhouser Bldg.
Lexington, KY 40506-0054
(606) 257-2000

Grambling State University
100 Main Street
Grambling, LA 71245
(318) 247-6941

Springfield College
Springfield, MA 01109
(413) 788-3136

Central Michigan University
Warriner 105
Mount Pleasant, MI 48859
(517) 774-3076

Michigan State University
East Lansing, MI 48824
(517) 355-8332

Mankato State University
Mankato, MN 56001
(507) 389-1822

University of Minnesota, Twin Cities
231 South Pillsbury Drive S.E.
240 Williamson Hall
Minneapolis, MN 55455
(612) 625-2008

University of Southern Mississippi
Southern Station Box 5011
Hattiesburg, MS 39406
(601) 266-5555

University of Missouri—Columbia
Columbia, MO 65211
(314) 882-7786

University of Nebraska at Omaha
Omaha, NE 68182
(402) 554-2393

University of New Hampshire
Durham, NH 03824
(603) 862-1360

Ithaca College
Danby Road
Ithaca, NY 14850
(607) 274-3124

State University of New York College at Brockport
Kenyon Street
Brockport, NY 14420
(716) 395-2751

State University of New York College at Cortland
P.O. Box 2000
Cortland, NY 13045
(607) 753-4711

East Carolina University
East Fifth Street
Greenville, NC 27858-4353
(919) 757-6640

University of North Carolina at Greensboro
1000 Spring Garden State
Greensboro, NC 27412
(919) 334-5243

University of North Carolina at Wilmington
601 South College Road
Wilmington, NC 28403-3297
(919) 395-3243

Oklahoma State University
104 Whitehurst Hall
Stillwater, OK 74078
(405) 774-6861

University of Oregon
Eugene, OR 97403
(503) 686-3201

Lincoln University
Lincoln University, PA 19352
(215) 932-8300

Pennsylvania State University
201 Shields Building
University Park, PA 16802
(814) 865-5471

Slippery Rock University of Pennsylvania
Slippery Rock, PA 16057
(412) 794-7203

Temple University
Broad Street and Montgomery Avenue
Philadelphia, PA 19122
(215) 787-7000

Clemson University
Clemson, SC 29634-4019
(803) 656-2287

University of North Texas
P.O. Box 13797
Denton, TX 76203
(817) 565-2681

Brigham Young University
Provo, UT 84602
(801) 378-2507

University of Utah
Salt Lake City, UT 84112
(801) 581-7281

Green Mountain College
Poultney, VT 05764
(802) 287-9313

Lyndon State College
Lyndonville, VT 05851
(802) 626-9371

Longwood College
Farmville, VA 23901
(804) 395-2060

Old Dominion University
Norfolk, VA 23529-0050
(804) 683-3637

Radford University
Radford, VA 24142
(703) 831-5371

Virginia Commonwealth University
910 West Franklin Street, Box 2526
Richmond, VA 23284
(804) 257-6124

Eastern Washington University
M.S. 148 Admissions Office
Cheney, WA 99004
(509) 359-2397

West Virginia University
Morgantown, WV 26506
(304) 766-3221

University of Wisconsin, LaCrosse
1725 State Street
LaCrosse, WI 54601
(608) 785-8067

The following colleges and universities offer a major in recreation therapy.

Mesa State College
P.O. Box 2647
Grand Junction, CO 81502
(303) 248-1376

Morris Brown College
634 Martin Luther King Drive
Atlanta, GA 30314
(404) 525-7831

College of St. Francis
500 Wilcox Street
Joliet, IL 60435
(815) 740-3400

Huntington College
Huntington, IN 46750
(219) 356-6000

Indiana Institute of Technology
1600 E. Washington Blvd.
Fort Wayne, IN 46803
(219) 422-5561, ext. 251

University of Southern Maine
37 College Avenue
Gorham, ME 04038
(207) 780-5215

Northeastern University
360 Huntington Avenue
Boston, MA 02115
(617) 437-2200

Grand Valley State University
College Landing
Allendale, MI 49401
(616) 985-2025

Lake Superior State University
1000 College Drive
Sault Sainte Marie, MI 49783
(906) 635-2231

College of Saint Mary
1901 South 72nd Street
Omaha, NE 68124
(402) 399-2405

Utica College of Syracuse University
Burrstone Road
Utica, NY 13502
(315) 792-3006

Belmont Abbey College
Belmont, NC 28012
(704) 825-3711

Catawba College
2300 West Innes Street
Salisbury, NC 28144
(704) 637-4402

Western Carolina University
Cullowhee, NC 28723
(704) 227-7317

Winston-Salem State University
Martin Luther King Drive
Winston-Salem, NC 27110
(919) 761-2070

Defiance College
701 North Clinton Street
Defiance, OH 43512
(419) 784-4010, ext. 359

York College of Pennsylvania
Country Club Road
York, PA 17403
(717) 846-7788

Texas Woman's University
P.O. Box 22909 TWU Station
Denton, TX 76204
(817) 898-3000

West Virginia State College
Institute, WV 25112
(304) 766-3221

BIOCHEMIST

The great majority of major colleges and universities, over 300 of them, offer concentrations in the field of biochemistry. Undergraduate degrees can be earned at all of these, and graduate degrees at many.